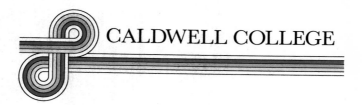

D1116698

POSITIVELY FALSE

POSITIVELY FALSE

Exposing the Myths around HIV and AIDS

Joan Shenton

Foreword by Gordon T. Stewart

I.B.Tauris
London · New York

Published in 1998 by
I.B.Tauris & Co. Ltd
Victoria House
Bloomsbury Square
London WC1B 4DZ

In the United States of America and Canada distributed by

St Martin's Press
175 Fifth Avenue
New York
NY 10010

A full CIP record for this book is available from the British Library
A full CIP record for this book is available from the Library of Congress

ISBN 1–86064–333–7
Library of Congress Catalog card number available

Copy-edited and laser-set by Oxford Publishing Services, Oxford

Printed and bound in Great Britain by WBC, Bridgend, Mid Glam.

'Men are so simple, and so much creatures of circumstance, that the deceiver will always find someone ready to be deceived.'
(Niccolò Machiavelli, *The Prince*, 1532)

This book is dedicated to all those who died
believing HIV would cause their death

Contents

Contents

Contents

Acronyms and Abbreviations

ACSUR   Association pour la coopération avec le Sud
AIDS   acquired immune deficiency syndrome
ATL   adult T-cell leukaemia
AZT   azidothymidine *or* zidovudine (generic name) *or* Retrovir (brand name)
BBC   British Broadcasting Corporation
BCC   Broadcasting Complaints Commission
BMA   British Medical Association
BMJ   *British Medical Journal*
CBL   Chester Beatty Laboratory
CDC   Center for Disease Control
CDS   Centres for Development of Health (Haiti)
CMV   cytomegalovirus
ddC   dideoxycytidine
ddI   dideoxyinosine
DMT   dimethyltryptamine (hallucinogenic drug)
DNA   deoxyribonucleic acid
EBV   Epstein–Barr virus
EIS   Epidemic Intelligence Service
ELISA   enzyme-linked immunosorbent assay
FDA   US Food and Drug Administration
GAG   Gays Against Genocide
GHESKIO   Haitian Group on Kaposi's Sarcoma and Opportunistic Infections
GRID   gay related immune deficiency
HEAL   Health Education AIDS Liaison
HIV   human immunodeficiency virus

HIV-SF	HIV-suppressive factors
HLA	human lymphocyte antigen
HTLV	human T-cell leukaemia virus
i.v.	intravenous
IBA	Independent Broadcasting Association
ICI	Imperial Chemical Industries
ICL	idiopathic CD4 lymphocytopaenia
INSERM	Institut national de Santé et de Recherche médicale
JAMA	*Journal of the American Medical Association*
JC	kind of virus
JIMHA	*Journal of the Interamerican Medical and Health Association*
KS	Kaposi's sarcoma
LAV	lymphadenopathy associated virus
LDK	recreational drug
LSE	London School of Economics and Political Science
MCA	Medicines Control Agency
MDA	methylenedioxyamphetamine
MDMA	methylenedioxymethylamphetamine (Ecstasy)
MP	Member of Parliament
MRC	Medical Research Council
MS	multiple sclerosis
NBA	National Basketball Association
NBC	National Broadcasting Company
NCI	National Cancer Institute
NEJM	*New England Journal of Medicine*
NIAID	National Institute of Allergy and Infectious Diseases
NIH	National Institutes of Health
NTSC	National Television System Committee
ORI	Office of Research Integrity
PBS	Public Broadcasting Service
PCP	pneumocystis carinii pneumonia *or* phencyclohexylpiperidine (the drug phencylidine; angel dust)
PCR	polymerase chain reaction
PDR	Physicians Desk Reference
PENTA	Paediatric European Network for Treatment in AIDS

PHLS	Public Health Laboratory Service
PI	protease inhibitor
PML	progressive multifocal leukoencephalopathy
PNAS	*Proceedings of the National Academy of Sciences*
RAID	Responsible AIDS Information at Dartmouth
RNA	ribonucleic acid
RTS	Royal Television Society
SCAM	Standing Committee on AZT Malpractice
SIV	simian immunodeficiency virus
SLE	systemic lupus erythematosus
SMON	subacute myelo-opticoneuropathy
STD	sexually transmitted disease
STP	hallucinogenic drug
T	thymus
T-cells	thymus matured lymphocytes (immune system cells)
TB	tuberculosis
UCL	University College London
UCLA	University of California at Los Angeles
UNICEF	United Nations Children's Fund
USAID	United States Agency for International Development
VA	Veterans' Administration
WHO	World Health Organization
YHC	recreational drug

Acknowledgements

I n a world where scientific and medical orthodoxies had closed their doors to inquiry, I thank those of its professions who kept their doors open for my questions: Professor Alfred Hässig, Dr Harvey Bialy, Professor Gordon Stewart, Dr Eleni Eleopulos, Dr Valendar Turner, Professor Fritz Ulmer, Professor Harry Rubin, Professor Charles Thomas, Professor Phillip Johnson, Mr Michael Freeman, Dr Fabio Franchi, Professor Beverly Griffin, Dr Stefan Lanka, Professor Kassi Manlan, Dr Martin Okot-Nwang, Dr Felix Konotey-Ahulu, Dr Andrew Herxheimer, and Dr Ricardo Leschot.

Thank you to David Lloyd, head of News and Current Affairs at Channel 4, his assistant editor Francesa O'Brien, and at an earlier stage Karen Brown, for making it possible to air the dissident debate and for their unflagging intellectual input. Thanks also to the Channel 4 lawyers headed by Don Christopher, including Jan Tomalin, Madeleine Sheahan and Mark Lambert for fighting our battles; to Christopher Griffin-Beale who looked after press and public relations for our first AIDS programme, and to Martin Stott who dealt with the rest, fending off the volley of insults after each programme with the greatest aplomb. I am very grateful also to Frank Riess and Professor Alfred Hässig for believing in me and supporting Meditel financially through the barren times. Also to the late Bill Bowie and the Bill Bowie Foundation for providing the finishing money for *Diary of an AIDS Dissident*. Thank you to Terrel Cass, head of the US Public Broadcasting Service channel WLIW, for keeping his word and broadcasting parts of the film in 'The Great AIDS Debate', and to lawyer Peter Smith who highlighted the injustice surrounding our Broadcasting Complaints Commission adjudication.

There are so many people who over the past ten years have encouraged, supported and nourished me through patches when it seemed difficult to sustain the assault against the AIDS orthodoxy: Mark Wood, Etsuro Totsuka, Gaby Berneck, Philip Barker and Julie Peakman; Sybil Duesberg, Jodie Schwartz, Jane Byrd, Bryan Ellison, Russell Schoch and David Rasnick in Berkeley; Michael Ellner and Frank Buianouckas from HEAL, New York; Simon Jenkins, Jane Balfour, Tony and Mary Mackintosh, Jackie and Kim Merino, Carol Wiseman, Corina Poore, Roberto Blandin, Astrid Luna, Dale Chalk, and my sister Rosemary Prior together with her husband the Revd David Prior. Thanks also to my nephew Daniel Prior who took me seriously enough to write about our work for his Edinburgh University newspaper; to Nick Fraser and Nik Gowing for telling me I should write this book; and to our Meditel team, Jad Adams, Felicity Milton, Nicky Hirsch, Melanie Wangler, Ian Owles, Jeremy Stavenhagen, Chris Renty and Pascal de Bock.

Thank you to the team at *Continuum* magazine, Huw Christie, Rafael Ramos, Tony Thompsett, Patrick Brough, Nigel Edwards, Chris Baker; and also to Alex Russell, Gareth James and James Whitehead for their generous help with research. In New York, Bob Guccione Jr and Celia Farber from *Spin* magazine and Charles Ortleb from the *New York Native* were always ready to help with moral support and information as were AIDS dissidents Kawi Schneider and Peter Schmidt and Peter Rath in Germany, Robert Laarhoven in Holland, Alfredo Embid in Spain, Michael Baumgartner in Switzerland and Ole Deraker in Sweden. On issues surrounding AIDS prejudice towards prostitutes I was greatly helped by Nina Lopez-Jones and Niki Adams of the English Collective of Prostitutes, and on drug trials involving babies from the black community Cristel Amiss of Black Women for Wages for Housework gave invaluable support.

Part of this book was written during my year in the Dominican Republic and there I thank Daniel Martinez and his family for their love and kindness, Prudencio (Papi) Martinez, Amarylis Tavares, Oneida Tavares, Elvira de la Rosa, Tomás Reyes, Kenny Padilla, Adri Reyes, Ana Ylda Martinez. And I thank Susanna Beutler for her good company, sense of humour and critical appraisal.

Enormous thanks go to Peter Duesberg for taking me by the scruff of the neck and leading me through a crash course in molecular biology

Acknowledgements

and to Dr Hector Gildemeister for being a constant friend and critic. Michael Verney-Elliott needs a very special thank you for patiently combing through the book and adding some of his own inimitable stylistic twists.

And finally thank you to my editor Iradj Bagherzade for beating me into shape through gentle persuasion.

Foreword

Joan Shenton is well known for her many appearances on various TV channels, on radio, in the press and in public meetings internationally. Until 1987, her prominence and reputation came from her journalistic expertise in exploring some major threats to health and medical problems, ranging from malnutrition to the toxicity of certain widely-used medicaments. Since then, she has focused her insight, immense energy and compassion on the suffering caused by the misunderstandings and deceptions which have arisen worldwide about AIDS.

My first meeting with her was about 1979 when she asked me to advise on a television programme about a toxic drug now withdrawn from use. This was the beginning of a period during which I served, along with other health professionals, as an adviser to the company Meditel which Joan founded. Joan has won a number of prestigious awards for open, accurate and informative communications via television and otherwise on health affairs. From frequent, outspoken sessions with her and her colleagues, whatever the topic, I grew to appreciate the quality of her commitment to the important new profession of medical journalism, which is now the source of awareness and often main stimulus to correction of contemporary hazards to health.

This was the track that led her into AIDS. Her experience made her doubt some of the certainties expressed about causation and treatment. When Peter Duesberg wrote his 1987 article on retroviruses at the invitation of the editor of *Cancer Research*, and stated that HIV could not cause AIDS, she was immediately interested, the more so when the article was ignored and then furiously repudiated by those who claimed to have discovered and worked with this new agent. Knowing that I had been working on epidemiological aspects of AIDS and other sexually transmitted diseases with the WHO, she called to ask my opinion. I approached some colleagues in the business to see what they thought of Duesberg's article. The response was that it was nonsense. The summit conference on AIDS in London in 1988 produced a consensus which endorsed that of an *ad hoc* meeting in Washington in 1984 and declared that HIV was sweeping by heterosexual transmission throughout the Americas, Europe, Australasia and the entire Third World to cause AIDS in a pandemic of unprecedented dimension and lethality. Experts and actuaries were predicting that this would cause millions of cases and hundreds of thousands of deaths within a few years.

Events since then have shown that most of these predictions were nonsensical and even fabricated. But the belief that general populations everywhere were at risk of AIDS from the spread of HIV by heterosexual transmission persisted in expert and official quarters, and was promulgated as undisputed fact to the general public by health authorities everywhere. Justifiable concern at local levels gave way to a panic internationally, fed by alarming estimates emanating mainly from a few sources in the USA and from the WHO, and from Third World countries where AIDS was viewed as a threat to survival of working populations. In the UK, the London Declaration led to a succession of apocalyptic warnings in all the media, exceeding only those of the World Health Organization, the US Centers for Disease Control and other health authorities notably, in the UK, of the Health Education Authority in its televised advertisements.

Any attempt to criticize any of this, even tentatively, was regarded as heresy or worse. But Joan Shenton and her small team, almost alone in the field of medical journalism, attempted just that, mainly in several programmes on Channel 4 television in the UK.

The book gives a candid account of what led to and followed this bold excursion into what had by then become the largest single issue in the history of medical science, replete with far more workers, publications, propaganda, prophecies, expenditure and political influence than any other issue. It is revealing as an insider document because it records responses and attitudes with good humour at the personal level. In this way, though at considerable cost to her enterprise, Joan Shenton has gained access to inner sanctums, and has punctured some inflated claims which are exempt at present from critical or indeed from any independent scrutiny.

In saying this, I do not exempt her from the same imperative, nor would she wish me to do so. In challenging medical and other ortho-doxies in this convoluted field, she is subject like the rest of us to judgements and interpretations with which many others would dis-agree. But her candour leaves her pages open to discussion if not correction of her robust views on the non-infectiousness of AIDS (regardless of HIV), of the situation in Africa and of the current chemotherapy. Even when I disagree with her, I can always see valid reasons for her vigorous defence of her views.

In the UK and many other industrialized countries, AIDS is far from being the disaster which was forecast. This book will help those who are interested or affected to understand why, and to be more realistic about the special pleadings which still outshout other medical priorities. It should rank as required reading for decision-makers because it offers insight into a continuing crisis in which some remarkable scientific discoveries and dedicated efforts have been confounded by misunderstandings, and by medical and political deceptions of the public on an unprecedented international scale.

Gordon T Stewart,
Emeritus Professor of Public Health,
University of Glasgow.

Preface: A False Hypothesis

The most formidable barrier to the advancement of science is the conventional wisdom of the dominant group.

(C. H. Waddington, geneticist 1905–75)

It was plain that he [Peter Duesberg] had a powerful scientific case to present. He is a very eminent scientist. And I was fascinated that the HIV establishment, as we call it now, absolutely refused to take it seriously. Their attitude was that we know that HIV causes AIDS. We decided that long ago. We settled it. Now we're doing research on that basis and just don't bother us. We don't want to hear about this doubt about our basic premise.

(Phillip E. Johnson, Professor of Law, University of California, Berkeley[1])

I t was in 1981 that the first cluster of cases of what was eventually to be called AIDS, was identified in five young homosexual men in California. They all had two medical conditions in common, a type of pneumonia called pneumocystis carinii pneumonia (PCP) and a form of blood vessel tumour called Kaposi's sarcoma (KS) causing internal and external lesions. They also had one other thing in common, they inhaled poppers – amyl and butyl nitrites. This drug was regularly used to enhance sexual pleasure and in particular to help dilate the anal orifice and allow 'fisting' (brachioproctal intercourse) in the aggressively promiscuous lifestyle of these particular young men.

The new-found sexual freedom that followed the gay liberation movement of the 1970s led some gay men into a fast track, high risk life-style, where drug-assisted sex became a necessary part of their daily life, and concomitant sexually transmitted diseases (STDs) were regarded as merely a recreational hazard easily put right with antibiotics.

It was in 1983 that 'HIV' was announced as 'the probable cause of AIDS' at a Washington press conference before any peer-reviewed papers had been published in a scientific journal.

The discovery of HIV and the panic over AIDS has led to over 100,000 published papers on HIV and AIDS. Some $40,000 million of the US taxpayers money and £2000 million in the UK has been spent on AIDS since 1984. Prevention programmes in the UK directed at the community as a whole, total over £500 million. Yet, in all this time, no cure for AIDS has been found and, despite their awareness of the need for 'safer sex', young gay men are still developing the AIDS syndrome.

Why? Because the AIDS edifice is built upon the false hypothesis that the retrovirus HIV is the cause of AIDS and that AIDS is an infectious disease. In fact, the AIDS syndrome has not behaved like an infectious disease would. It has remained restricted to certain high risk groups (which will be described later); groups that are already prone to severe immune suppression.

As long ago as 1986, molecular biologist Professor Peter Duesberg of the University of California at Berkeley, began his assault on the AIDS orthodoxy by stating his reasons why HIV cannot kill cells and cannot therefore be pathogenic, or cause death. Just because HIV is said to be present in most cases of AIDS does not mean it is the cause.

'Association does not prove causation,' says Duesberg. AIDS, he says, is not an infectious disease. As a respected scientist in the field of retrovirology he was listened to briefly at first and then quickly dismissed by his peers. The AIDS research roller coaster was far too lucrative for it to be stopped in its tracks by a single dissenting voice, and plague terror had already gripped governments and people. Why was there only one voice, you may ask? Well, Copernicus, Galileo and Columbus stood alone in their beliefs – and were proved right in the end (although it took 350 years for Galileo's heresy to be pardoned by the relevant Vatican committees).

This book will chronicle our challenge over the last ten years to the firmly held belief that HIV causes AIDS, and the orthodoxy's response to that challenge. It will describe the relationships between scientists like

Robert Gallo and Luc Montagnier, catapulted to fame and fortune by their AIDS research, and Peter Duesberg who dared to oppose them. The rivalries, jealousies and deceits woven into the Byzantine politics of the most highly financed laboratories in the world will be unravelled.

In 1987 we set out to tell the story of how Peter Duesberg, who had himself been the first scientist to map the genetic sequence of retro-viruses, threw down the gauntlet to the AIDS establishment.

Not only does Duesberg maintain that HIV cannot cause AIDS, he puts forward the hypothesis that the breakdown of the immune system, described as the AIDS syndrome, is caused by long-term recreational and intravenous drug use and certain clinical conditions requiring immune-suppressant blood transfusions or, as in haemophilia, anticoagulant blood clotting factors. The ensuing toxic overload allows opportunistic infections to take over the undefended body.

In the very early days of AIDS, the toxic hypothesis was thought to be an important causal factor. The first 'cluster' of gay men with 'AIDS' symptoms in California had all used poppers (amyl and butyl nitrite inhalants), to enhance sexual pleasure and assist anal intercourse. Their condition was originally described as GRID – gay related immune deficiency. But as soon as HIV appeared on the scene, the toxic hypothesis was dropped and the virus/AIDS hypothesis was embraced with enthusiasm both by the medical orthodoxy and the gay community.

This book will dig into our extensive archive and record the triumphs and frustrations of those people, including other well-known scientists, health professionals, people with AIDS, and many gay and straight men and women, who dared challenge this same AIDS establishment. It will describe the way our small independent television production company, Meditel, started out on its first documentary on the subject, confident that we could reshape people's thinking about AIDS – not knowing then how the scientific establishment would close ranks against us. However, over a period of ten years we have been able to keep the subject alive with the help of David Lloyd, editor of the *Dispatches* series at Channel 4 Television who commissioned four documentaries from us, and was later to develop a fifth; Joanne Sawicki, features editor at Sky News, who transmitted four shorter reports on the subject and Terrel Cass, head of the American PBS

Channel WLIW New York who bought our footage and flew us over for a two-hour discussion programme. The AIDS debate has taken over our lives and led us into one of the most exciting scientific debates of the century.

In the course of making our documentaries we travelled across the USA seven times on research and filming trips interviewing scores of both orthodox and dissident scientists as well as people with AIDS. We also filmed extensively in Europe and travelled through six countries in East and West Africa. The book is structured around the making of those programmes between 1989 and 1997. The research surrounding them grew, as did the arguments between the key scientists, as we completed one programme and went on to the next.

What I have learned over these years is that the scientific community is no longer free. Today science can be bought, and the individual dissenting voice is able to be silenced and dismissed because of the enormous sums of money involved in protecting a prevailing hypothesis, however flawed it may be. Politics, power and money dominate the scientific research field to such an extent that it is now no longer possible to put a hypothesis that has become dogma to the test. Scientific trials sponsored by pharmaceutical companies often involve many different university faculties at one time and consequently tie up most of the expert voices. The dogma is written up in tablets of stone in medical textbooks and young science students swallow it without question. Those that are already in well paid jobs find it easier not to rock the boat. What would be the point? They would simply lose their jobs.

Duesberg has his own explanation on the puzzle as to why the dogma of the current AIDS hypothesis remains sacrosanct:

Why doesn't a young ambitious scientist make a name for himself by questioning it? The answer lies in the strong conformist pressures on scientists, particularly young, untenured scientists, in the age of biotechnology. Their conceptual obedience to the establishment is maintained by controlled access to research grants, journals and positions, and rewarded by conference engagements, personal prizes, consultantships [sic], stocks and co-ownership in companies. A dissenter would have to be truly independent and prepared for a variety of sanctions.[2]

Preface: A False Hypothesis

The editors of the book *Research Fraud in the Behavioural and Biomedical Sciences* put it this way, 'The commercialism of academia ... and a market mentality to research has led to anti-intellectualism and dishonesty.'[3] The HIV test kit patents, the profits from the so-called anti-AIDS drug azidothymidine (AZT), and the flow of government funds made available for vaccine research and AIDS prevention have led to a consensus collusion surrounding AIDS that could take decades to dismantle. It may even need 'dead men's shoes' before the younger generation of scientists finds the courage and confidence to look into the last decade of bad science surrounding AIDS research. So bad has been the science that Dr Harvey Bialy, scientific editor of *Bio/Technology* (sister journal to *Nature*) and friend of Peter Duesberg has consistently refused to publish the majority of HIV related papers submitted to his journal.

The reactions to Duesberg's publications and to our reflection of his work have been vicious. The orthodoxy decided to close ranks against him, and his views are simply not discussed in the scientific journals. The key justification from leading members of the orthodoxy for stamping on any challenge to the virus/AIDS hypothesis has been that if the HIV = AIDS = death hypothesis is eventually proved correct, then lending a platform to the dissident view will have caused untold damage.

But herein lies the enormous culpability of an orthodoxy that attempts to stamp out dissent. For, in the absence of reliable clinical evidence for the HIV = AIDS = death hypothesis, it remains just that – a hypothesis. The advancement of science has always been based on postulating alternative hypotheses and then putting them to the test. By stifling dissenting views, the orthodoxy can be held responsible for far greater damage, if those dissenting views are eventually proved to be right, because research will have been misdirected over a very long period of time and credibility in scientific method will have been totally undermined.

By definition, no tenable hypothesis can be eliminated until scientific evidence establishes where the truth lies. Until that time, tenable hypotheses should be able to compete with each other in an open field of intelligent and sensible discourse and debate. By stifling discourse and debate on dissenting views the orthodoxy is engaged in the unpardonable scientific sin of blocking off legitimate inquiry into a hypothesis that may itself become the future orthodox view. In the meanwhile, millions in research funding and energy will have been misdirected. So, in a curious way the orthodox attempt at a moral argument against giving dissidents a platform for fear of distracting research, has its mirror image in the dissident view. If the orthodox hypothesis is proved wrong, by stifling the dissidents, the orthodoxy will become morally responsible for the damage caused by the misdirecting of research efforts in search of the right answer.

Although Duesberg's first paper criticising the HIV = AIDS hypothesis was published in a major science journal, *Cancer Research*[4] and, with difficulty, a further paper in the *Proceedings of the National Academy of Sciences (PNAS)*,[5] journals like *Nature* have repeatedly turned down his papers. Its ex-editor, Sir John Maddox, has allowed only a few hundred-word replies from Duesberg after publishing 2000-word articles attacking him both personally and professionally. The degree of censorship in the scientific and lay press has been astonishing and will be dealt with in these pages.

The Medical Research Council, the European Union, the World Health Organization, the US National Institutes of Health and Centers for Disease Control, all locked into massive AIDS programmes, have allowed institutional money to be wasted in their stubborn adherence to the virus-AIDS hypothesis. They have created elite AIDS cadres wandering nomadically from one international AIDS conference to another, grazing on yet another set of incomprehensible statistics on the alleged spread of HIV.

Duesberg has been joined in his struggle against the AIDS orthodoxy by other scientists, notably 500 scientists and health professionals who have formed the Group for the Scientific Reappraisal of the HIV/AIDS Hypothesis. One of its members is Dr Kary Mullis. Nobel prize winner for chemistry in 1993 and inventor of a highly sensitive method used to identify HIV, he says:

I can't find a single virologist who will give me references which show that HIV is the probable cause of AIDS. On an issue as important as this, there should be a set of scientific documents somewhere, research papers written by people who are accessible, demonstrating this. But they are not available. If you ask a virologist for that information you don't get an answer, you get fury.[6]

But it is not only virologists and government bodies who have perpetrated the myth of HIV. 'Compassionate celebrity' as journalist Chris Dunkley described it, has had an enormous part to play, 'with film stars and disc jockeys adopting deeply concerned expressions as they roll condoms on to their fingers'.[7]

This compassionate celebrity approach has never been better performed than by my childhood heroine, film star Elizabeth Taylor, at Wembley Stadium in her tribute to the rock star Freddie Mercury. It was common knowledge that Mercury had abused drugs heavily over many years, but so entrenched had the 'infectious HIV virus' hypothesis become with its alleged sexual path towards AIDS, that Taylor glossed over any drug risks. Addressing herself to 'teenagers' and 'young adults', she said:

You are the future of our world. You are the best and brightest. . . . Protect yourselves! Every time you have sex, use a condom. Every single time. Straight sex, gay sex, bisexual sex. Use a condom whoever you are. And if you use drugs, don't share the needle. Protect yourself. Love yourself. Respect yourself. Because I will keep telling you until you do. And I won't give in because the world needs you to live. We love you. We care.[8]

'And if you use drugs, don't share the needle', Taylor had said. Apparently it was all right to pump yourself with drugs as long as you did not share the needles. It was the virus that caused AIDS so only the needles seemed to matter, not what went through them. Only the condoms were important, not the disease-linked promiscuity that might go with them.

So What is HIV?

The human immunodeficiency virus belongs to a comparatively recently identified group of viruses known as retroviruses, which are considered to be unique members of the virus family of pathogens (disease-causing agents).

All viruses are pirates.[9] They invade, pillage, destroy and sometimes take up residence in their target vessel. Viruses are pieces of genetic material wrapped up inside a protein coat. They are made of DNA (deoxyribonucleic acid) or RNA (ribonucleic acid). Most viruses are made of DNA, which is a double-stranded molecule containing, in a chemically coded form, all the information needed to build, control and maintain a living organism. DNA is, in fact, our genetic blueprint.

Some viruses are made of RNA. A minority of these are called retroviruses and HIV is one of them. Current orthodoxy maintains that retroviruses like HIV, made of RNA, are single stranded and when they enter a new cell, need the DNA of their host cell in order to survive. They can be described as cell dependent scavengers.

The more common DNA viruses are like hand-grenades in a plastic pouch. Inside each hand-grenade is a full set of instructions on how the virus can copy itself and, when it multiplies, how to pass the genetic information on to the new cells. So, when the hand-grenade enters a cell, it makes copies of itself until the cell is ready to burst like a ripe seedpod. The destroyed host cell then spills out all the perfectly formed new hand-grenades, hungry to go off and infect other cells.

Retroviruses, like other viruses, need their host cell in order to stay alive but have to transform their RNA into DNA before they can knit themselves into the host cell's DNA. This chemical process makes use of an enzyme called reverse transcriptase, enabling the retrovirus to knit its RNA into the DNA – the genetic heart – of the cell it is invading, where it quietly takes up residence and lies dormant. Once the retrovirus has integrated itself with its host, it is called a 'provirus'. Should that cell divide, it will carry its integrated passenger provirus with it and may shed some particles on the way.

These theories were widely believed in 1983 when HIV was first posited to be the cause of AIDS. HIV then acquired a malign, almost mystical talismanic quality. However, it was soon pointed out that retroviruses are very common and indeed most cellular blueprints of mammals contain many different ones, sometimes running to hundreds, which apparently lie dormant like so many burnt out microchips.

So a retrovirus is much less active than an ordinary virus and will lie passively inside the nucleus of the host cell, appearing to do nothing. For this reason retroviruses have been described as gentle, lazy and benign, so much so that, in the view of Peter Duesberg and now many other scientists, HIV cannot cause AIDS.

Today an even more radically heretical position about AIDS is being expressed by scientists in Perth (Western Australia), Germany and Switzerland. They maintain that HIV has never been isolated. It is usually identified through finding the presence of antibodies to mixed proteins (ELISA test) or separated proteins (Western blot test), said to be specific to HIV. However, these proteins are in all of us and our antibodies to them can become dramatically raised when the body is under severe immune stress. Other ways of identifying HIV involve amplifying the genetic content of the retrovirus through PCR (polymerase chain reaction). But, say these scientists, what is being found are genetic fragments or debris, not a whole virus capable of going on to infect another cell. This is what is mistakenly being called HIV they say. HIV itself does not exist.

It is always hard for new and controversial views to get an airing when the orthodoxy becomes entrenched, as is the case with AIDS. We shall see below how the peer review process exercised by science journals can effectively exclude competing hypotheses. This is where the London-based journal *Continuum* has played an important role in publishing a steady stream of papers from the above scientists when they have been repeatedly rejected by orthodox journals.[10]

The theory that HIV has never been isolated and is being wrongly identified puts the whole of the HIV testing machinery into question. The test itself, say this group of scientists, is invalid because there is no gold standard (no actual virus) to measure against.

We have put this theory to the test for a Channel 4 *Dispatches* programme and have some sensational results. We have discovered inconsistencies between the different test kits on the market, and have found that individuals testing HIV positive one week have tested negative one month later. In addition, people with raised proteins in their blood from rheumatic or autoimmune conditions have tested HIV positive when they had no AIDS-defining diseases.

This is not the first time that medical science has got it wrong. Contagion mania – the desire to blame an exogenous infectious agent for a disease has led to some horrifying situations in the past. Take two examples, the pellagra plague and SMON (subacute myelo-optic neuropathy).

False: The Story of Pellagra

It took 15 years for the lone voice of Dr Joseph Goldberger to be heeded about pellagra. Since the eighteenth century, this condition had affected poor communities in Europe, which suffered from a niacin (vitamin B) deficiency due to a corn-based diet that almost completely excluded other vegetables. Maize had been the staple diet in the Americas for millennia, and the pre-Columbian inhabitants did not contract pellagra, for they had learnt how to extract the essential vitamin B from the corn during its preparation. But this culinary art was lost to other civilizations.

Although pellagra did not spread beyond its risk groups, a classic indicator of a non-infectious disease, and never affected nursing staff, many doctors pronounced it a contagious bacterial disease. Patients with the disease developed terrible skin lesions, nerve damage, dementia, diarrhoea, wasting syndrome and finally died. Sailors with symptoms of the condition were thrown off ships for fear that they would infect the rest of the crew, and when a huge outbreak occurred in poor farming communities in the southern states of America, patients were isolated in mental asylums and in prisons. By 1914, 200,000 cases were reported. It was then that Dr Goldberger was brought in to head a special commission.

When Goldberger visited the south and ventured into the rural areas and mental asylums, he noticed something that had escaped the microbe hunters, such was their frenzy to find an infectious agent. He noticed that none of the people closest to the pellagra victims, their doctors and their nurses, had caught the disease. He also noticed that the two groups were eating entirely different diets. The health workers were eating fresh fruit and vegetables and the farmers their customary corn diet.[11] Goldberger concluded that a nutritional deficiency was the cause of pellagra. In a striking parallel with the AIDS story, his findings were greeted with alarm and anger by those committed to the contagious hypothesis. Doctors joined together to criticize him and his theories were ridiculed. He became so exasperated that in a dramatic bid to prove that pellagra was not infectious he, his wife and 14 co-workers injected themselves with samples of blood, mucous and other bodily fluids from pellagra patients. None contracted the disease. Even this spectacular demonstration did not change the prevailing view, and people with pellagra continued to die. Niacin, the vitamin missing in the diet of people with pellagra was finally isolated in the mid-1930s, five years after Goldberger's death.[12]

False: The Story of SMON

Similarly, in the 1960s and 1970s a mysterious disease afflicted many thousands of people in Japan; it was called SMON (subacute myelo-optic neuropathy). It caused paralysis, blindness and death. In the space of a few years 700 people died and 11,000 severely nerve-damaged victims formed a support group. Fearing an infectious agent, the Japanese health authorities were concerned that the forthcoming Olympic Games in Japan might be affected. A virus called the 'Inoue SMON virus', named after one of the scientists investigating the disease, was blamed. Many victims committed suicide fearing they would contaminate their relatives; others died of sheer fright.

Fortunately, the Japanese government decided to fund a multidisciplinary committee to research into the problem. No longer could the virologists and infectologists hold sway. Some good old-fashioned observational science came into play and the detective work of Professor Tadeo Tsubaki tracked the problem down to an adverse reaction caused by long-term use of a common anti-diarrhoeal drug called Entero-Vioform, containing clioquinol.

The problem was simply one of toxicity – there was no infectious agent. Other cases were found in Sweden, Australia, the UK and the USA. Thousands of Japanese victims took their case to court. After a nine-year struggle and some remarkably tenacious legal work from, in particular, a young Japanese international human rights lawyer Etsuro

Totsuka, who brought the issue under an international spotlight, Ciba-Geigy the manufacturers of Entero-Vioform had to pay more than £350 million in compensation. In the end, several hundred lawyers became involved and the whole painful process had taken 15 years.[13]

It is interesting to note that this problem would not have been resolved within the scientific community. The powerful hold of pharmaceutical company interests had skilfully silenced the few dissenting voices who supported the toxic hypothesis. It was only when litigation started that the actual scientific facts came to light, and the extent of the damage and human suffering became known. Ciba-Geigy never accepted liability but eventually withdrew the sale of Entero-Vioform and other clioquinol-based products as antidiarrhoeals around the world.

There are many other significant parallels that can be drawn from the above examples when it comes to the debate about HIV and AIDS. An important factor to bear in mind is that the notion that HIV causes AIDS has never been anything more than an unproven hypothesis. The ultimate measure of the accuracy of any hypothesis is the fulfilment of predictions based upon it. Not one of the predictions for AIDS based on the spread of HIV has come true. In the United States, according to Center for Disease Control (CDC) figures, the estimated number of people with HIV has remained static over the last ten years at one million and, paradoxically, has even dropped to 800,000 more recently. Government predictions in the USA and UK for the number of AIDS cases have been consistently wrong. There has, in fact been no epidemic – entirely the reverse. Figures for AIDS have been dropping, but you would not know it because the CDC's AIDS statistics are published cumulatively, dating back to the early 1980s. What the public never knows is that the percentage of new AIDS cases has been decreasing steadily over the last few years, and that there has been no actual annual incremental increase in AIDS cases (comparing year with year) over the last ten years. But then, since when did shrinking figures for an alleged pandemic persuade government research funders to open up their coffers?

In fact, 'HIV disease' and AIDS as we know them have remained firmly locked into clearly defined high risk groups, namely homosexual men, long-term recreational drug users, intravenous drug users, athletes and sportsmen using performance-enhancing drugs, and people in clinical risk groups like recipients of blood transfusions and haemophiliacs taking 99 per cent impure clotting Factor VIII. But political correctness has been a further obstacle in the path towards opening up the AIDS debate. Pointing a finger at the lifestyle of some gay men and drug users has raised sensitivities. Better to stick to the 'virus from hell' hypothesis than to focus on a group that had suffered discrimination for so many years and was now emerging into a world of gay liberation. Any arguments that singled out these groups were immediately labelled as homophobic and belonging to the far right of the political spectrum.

Apart from the high risk groups mentioned above, all other reported cases of AIDS have to be seen in the light of the way AIDS is officially defined. From the first two defining diseases, Kaposi's sarcoma and pneumocystis carinii pneumonia, observed in the group of Californian men mentioned earlier, the basis for the diagnosis of AIDS has been stretched from year to year to include 29 widely differing defining illnesses from diarrhoea to dementia, culminating in pulmonary tuberculosis, which thereby includes most of sub-Saharan Africa, and cervical cancer, adding more women to the overall AIDS figures. When HIV is present, the diagnosis is AIDS and when HIV is absent, it's simply the old disease. This periodic moving of the goal posts offers free rein for extensive misdiagnosis, compounded by the fact that at least half of the reported cases of AIDS are based on a presumptive clinical diagnosis, not backed up by an HIV test.

Building upon a false hypothesis is like building a house on sand. It will stand up for a while and then break into pieces. The AIDS edifice is not only built on sand, it houses closed minds and has closed its doors to scrutiny. The inexorable death sentence – 'you have ten years at most' pronounced by doctors on young men and women has led to some of the most intense human suffering imaginable. It has broken up families, alienated individuals from their communities and led to psychological death and suicide.

There is absolutely no doubt that the arguments put forward by those challenging the virus/AIDS hypothesis have not been properly addressed. Blatant censorship has prevented any intelligent debate. The time has now come to open up that debate and to describe the making of what author John Lauritsen, who has emerged as one of the articulate spokesmen on the dissident view of AIDS, describes as 'the most colossal blunder in medical history'.

Chapter 1

Journey into Dissidence

The Lupus Experience

T he journey that led me to question the perceived wisdom on HIV and AIDS began in July 1972 on a balmy holiday in northern Spain. I had developed diarrhoea in England before leaving for Spain. It deteriorated in Spain and I was admitted to hospital in northern Spain where the doctors thought I had cholera. I was given a cocktail of drugs, which, combined with the sulphonamide drugs I had bought over the counter, caused a massive drug cross-reaction. I began to develop symptoms of a life-threatening condition called drug-induced systemic lupus erythematosus (SLE). I flew back to London and was admitted to Westminster Hospital. My weight plunged to under 40 kilos, I developed rashes that spread all over my body, my liver and the lining of my heart became inflamed and I had massive convulsions. I did nearly die, and have a hazy memory of a distraught nurse in tears trying to feel my pulse and then whispering, 'She's going.'

It was cortisone (a corticosteroid) that saved my life but the very high initial dose of 80 milligrams a day caused me to become a 'steroid patient'. I put on weight, developed a 'moon face' and one of my hip joints began to crumble. After three years on a walking stick, I scoured Britain to find a surgeon who would give me a hip replacement. They all said I was too young. Finally, I came across orthopaedic surgeon Michael Freeman. Using an experimental technique he had developed

1

for younger people, he provided a total hip replacement which completely restored my mobility.

My illness led to my losing my job as a presenter on BBC *Nationwide*, but after a year of convalescence, I returned to television and began to specialize in medical stories. My focus was on injury from prescribed drugs, which meant tackling some of the most powerful pharmaceutical companies in the world – Ciba-Geigy, Imperial Chemical Industries (ICI), Hoechst and Squibb.

With my independent production company, Meditel Productions, we were to go on to make over 100 documentaries and to win seven international awards. But this was only the beginning.

In 1982, together with my co-directors Alison Hawkes and Jad Adams, we produced our first series for Channel 4 on drug injury, called *Kill or Cure?*, under the guidance of pharmacologist Dr Andrew Herxheimer. This six-part series described some of the worst drug injury disasters, including the story of SMON (described in the preface). *Kill or Cure?* was screened in many different countries and was eventually used by University College London Medical School in its pharmacology courses.

There followed many more stories. We tracked the dumping of dangerous medicines in Third World countries. We challenged the validity of the campaign to lower the population's cholesterol levels through dietary change. We criticized the indiscriminate use of exogenous hormones in women, like the pill (when started very young) and the enthusiasm for hormone replacement therapy – both of which increase the risk of breast cancer. None of these stories has made us popular with the powerful pharmaceutical industry and its disciples in the field of medicine, but thankfully some editors and TV channels were willing to air these 'difficult' issues.

Taking on the AIDS Debate

When the AIDS story broke dramatically in the world's press, I thought we should leave it alone. Many competent medical and science journalists had taken up the cause and there seemed no role for our type of investigative, behind the scenes, work.

What led us to change our minds is described below. But when we did eventually take the subject on, it led to a decade of furious research and seven television documentaries. Somehow AIDS was different. It took our small investigative team by surprise. With all the other subjects we had tackled there was a specific focus and a specific outcome. I thought AIDS would be the same – that by pointing out the flaws in the science that said AIDS was infectious and caused by a single virus that we would at least open up a debate and bring about a shift in opinion. Not a bit of it.

I entered the AIDS debate with a certain journalistic campaigning innocence and zeal. Gradually, I began to realize that the wall of opposition was unbreachable. We were up against massive collusion between a dogmatic scientific establishment and sheepish governments being bullied into handing over thousands of millions of dollars to further research into a bogus and unproven hypothesis. This, combined with a pseudo-religious belief in an all-pervading infectious virus promoted by a highly politicized lobby that wanted to believe in the virus from hell, was a devastating force. We were undeterred, even though my own peers saw me as a person obsessed with the subject. Perhaps I was and still am, but when one has accumulated a body of knowledge and is faced with facts that defy explanation in the context of orthodox thinking, when it becomes clear that minds are closed, that the very essence of scientific thought and discourse is being subverted, the frustration can be overwhelming. But in my case, it has felt more like drowning. The harder I tried, the more sceptical and unbelieving anyone in a position to commission our work became.

Instead of giving up, we continued to buzz like gnats around our opponents. We did this through the letters pages of national newspapers, by barraging TV news and current affairs editors with proposals, by approaching friendly MPs like George Galloway who asked a series of questions in the House, and by organizing demonstrations outside hospitals promoting trials of the so-called AIDS drug AZT (azidothymidine). We even protested, outside the Medical Research Council (MRC), demanding to be allowed to see the raw data surrounding toxicity after the AZT Concorde trial. (More on these 'trials' later.)

Nothing would budge. Eight years after entering the AIDS debate in 1987, my initial zeal and enthusiasm had turned into a streetwise cynicism and at one point a sense of despair set in. 'Try another subject,' my friends told me. And I did. I plunged into the dangers of the pill and breast cancer[1] and into an investigation into cot deaths and their association with toxic fire retardant chemicals in mattresses[2] – all solid material for leading current affairs programmes. But every day more and more phone calls came in with more and more inside information about AIDS. And then the avalanche of requests for scripts and documents set it. Every week we received letters and calls from abroad – from doctors (some HIV positive), medical students, network television and radio researchers and fellow AIDS campaigners. Our office, tucked away at the back of a large building in Covent Garden, in London, had become a community centre and meeting point for scores of HIV positive men, thirsty for information and reassurance – and our business had turned itself into a charitable foundation.

By 1989, Jad Adams, who two years earlier had made our first film about *AIDS: The Unheard Voices*, had gone off to write a hefty biography of Tony Benn, the politician. That left Felicity Milton, Nicky Hirsch and me to research, write proposals and run the office, and Michael Verney-Elliott and biochemist Dr Hector Gildemeister to continue with their daily discourse on the AIDS debate.

Michael and Hector are what might be described as conservative gay men. Michael, in his fifties but looking many years younger, had come to us first and triggered our earliest investigations into the subject. His caustic wit and verbal agility kept us all on our toes. He had an enormous breadth of knowledge – antiques collector, actor, television drama producer and now AIDS. He decided to teach himself the basics of virology and molecular biology and could carry on the most sophisticated conversations with scientists in the field.

Hector I had known since Oxford days. He is a biochemist, tall and distinguished with silver grey hair. He had heard we were questioning the role of HIV and walked back into my life with the insatiable curiosity of a man who wanted to know if he was at risk of AIDS. As he began his own lines of inquiry, his sense of incredulity at the enormity of 'the mistake' about AIDS was always refreshing, as was the animated and frequently vitriolic sparring that went on daily between him and Michael.

Added to our team came Pascal de Bock, a slim Belgian theatre charge nurse at a London teaching hospital. He had diabetes and when the HIV death sentence was pronounced upon him, he was shocked and afraid. He had to leave his job (in case he contaminated surgery patients – although there has never been a documented case of this in the history of AIDS). He decided to work with us as a volunteer for over a year. He was very striking in his T-shirt and jeans, swathed in oriental jewellery, pale face and severely shaven head. Pascal had been put on AZT but it made him very ill and he had a stroke. He decided to throw away all his medicines, joined a group called Positively Healthy, found a new lover, Paul, set up house with him and his health has improved ever since. No more bronchitis, no more skin problems, no more general malaise. In fact, he ended up looking fit, fatter and altogether well.

Cass Mann would drop in at intervals looking flamboyant. He had founded Positively Healthy, a support group with hundreds of HIV positive members, and with his whiplash tongue was always at the ready with an acidic quip, usually at the expense of fellow gays wedded to the virus/AIDS hypothesis.

This was the team that was to plunge into battle about HIV and AIDS with vigour over the next few years, never guessing how, little by little, the enormity of the AIDS cover-up would envelop us. The more we delved, the more we discovered the darker side of some of the world's scientists, and the ruthlessness and dishonesty that can surround 'high science'.

Chapter 2

'AIDS: The Unheard Voices'

Bad Blood: Could it Cause AIDS?

It was November 1986 when one of my closest friends, Carol Wiseman, who is a television drama director, rang me. She was working with drama producer Michael Verney-Elliott on a London Weekend Television production. 'Can you speak to Michael?' She said. 'He is completely consumed with his ideas about AIDS. He says there's something terribly wrong and I'm not in a position to judge.'

I arranged to meet Verney-Elliott for lunch. When he arrived he was staggering under the weight of a huge briefcase stuffed with medical research papers. He was carrying two years of research on his back. Lunch went on for three hours while he piled one paper after another on the table. 'Nothing on AIDS adds up. Here is a circumscribed epidemic which appears to have originated in a specific group of people,' he said. 'But where does it come from?' Verney-Elliott had plunged into his investigations propelled by anger that gay men were being blamed for spreading AIDS. 'They are blaming gay men for spreading the disease from Africa and Haiti through sex, but I think it's got more to do with damage to the immune system from blood contaminated with impurities that are being illegally imported from Third World countries where people are very sick.' Verney-Elliott felt that looking more closely at HIV positive haemophiliacs might give us a clue, and he had already contacted several leading haemophilia experts to sound out their views and voice his own disquiet.

'But there's another thing that doesn't tally,' he said. 'Why was AIDS first identified in a group of gay men in California who all had Kaposi's sarcoma, a very specific type of skin cancer and PCP [pneumocystis carinii pneumonia], a very unusual type of pneumonia? These cases are very different from the AIDS-haemophilia situation.'

I went back to the office with my head reeling, and discussed the meeting with my colleague, producer Jad Adams, who had been working closely with me on our medical programmes for the past four years. Adams agreed to have further discussions with Michael Verney-Elliott himself. I am not quite sure whether we adopted Verney-Elliott or whether he adopted us, but he moved in. Adams, Verney-Elliott and I spent many hours talking through the anomalies surrounding HIV and AIDS. The two of them focused on the contaminated blood theory and the first investigations on our fateful AIDS journey were underway.

They discovered that a company called Hemo-Caribbean had signed a contract with Haiti's 'Papa Doc' Duvalier just before he died in 1971, which would allow the company to extract plasma from Haitians for a term of ten years. Hemo-Caribbean were able to operate for some 18 months, from a building in the Rue des Remparts, Port au Prince, buying plasma for $3 to $5 per donation, before Papa Doc's son 'Baby Doc' Duvalier closed it down in November 1972 following an outcry that the drug companies were draining the life blood from the poor for profit. In all, some 75,000 litres of plasma were shipped to the USA, imported by four major pharmaceutical companies for processing into blood products albumen, gammaglobulin, immuno-globulin, Factors 8 and 9 and laboratory diagnostics. Adams and Verney-Elliott also found out about the illegal exportation of plasma from Brazil, the frozen bags being labelled 'orange juice'. Yet another company was allegedly flying Third World blood plasma into Montreal's Mirabel Airport, relabelling it 'made in Canada' and rerouting it to Europe.

Screening of blood donors and heat treatment of plasma products to 'clean them up' became mandatory in 1985. This meant that all blood donors had to be checked for various infectious agents such as hepatitis B and, as many people thought, HIV. Heat treatment of the plasma products would act as a double safety check to kill off any viruses and impurities that may have got through the screening process. The screening and heat treatment was therefore useful (regardless of whether HIV was the cause of AIDS) as it helped to reduce harmful agents in the blood products.

Whether toxic effects resulting from the importation and use of dirty blood from poor donors in the Third World, and from drug addicts and other sick people in the USA who sold blood to help finance their addiction, played a role in the escalating AIDS figures before the 1985 precautionary measures were introduced is not known. But in 1987, before we had read Peter Duesberg's first paper challenging HIV as the cause of AIDS, we felt it was worth investigating. So did David Lloyd, editor of Channel 4's *Dispatches*. He gave us development money for the 'Bad Blood' project and Adams and Verney-Elliott set off for the United States and Canada to research the subject.

Discovering Duesberg:
The Leading AIDS Dissident Academic

When they came back, Adams presented me with two separate projects – the blood story and a completely new angle on the AIDS story. It was impossible now to get definitive proof of the 'orange-juice' plasma story. No one wanted to talk about this disreputable trade in Third World blood and it was not possible actually to get hold of a relabelled sample, so the bad blood story had to be abandoned. However, during the research trip, Adams and Verney-Elliott had met with many scientists who were convinced that HIV could not be the sole cause of AIDS. What influenced Adams most was a paper by a distinguished German virologist now teaching and doing research at the University of California. Peter Duesberg's paper, 'Retroviruses as carcinogens and pathogens: expectations and reality', published in *Cancer Research*, elegantly questioned the role of retroviruses in caus-ing cancer and the role of HIV in AIDS. Here was a respected scientist plausibly arguing that the perceived wisdom on AIDS was not on the right track. Adams, Verney-Elliott and I decided on their return – fate-fully as it turned out – that it was important to give voice to these dissenters.

Peter Duesberg was no fringe scientist. He was a well-established molecular biologist at Berkeley, University of California, who had pioneered retrovirus research and led the team that mapped the genetic sequence of the retrovirus. He had also been the first scientist to isolate a cancer gene and in 1971 had been honoured as California Scientist of the Year. To his laurels he had added election to the prestigious National Academy of Scientists and an Outstanding Investigator Grant from the US National Institutes of Health (NIH). Duesberg was also well known for turning the spotlight on to significant gaps in the understanding of current scientific orthodoxies. And most interestingly he had cemented his integrity as a scientist by daring to challenge the very orthodoxy he had helped to establish. He questioned the then fashionable view that retroviruses (the RNA viruses that depend on their host cell because they need their host cell's DNA in order to survive) could cause cancer.

We needed no persuading to focus on Duesberg's challenge to the received wisdom on AIDS, so we presented a completely new outline to David Lloyd at Channel 4. Visiting David always reminded me of my university tutorials. There he sat with his monk-like fringe chopped across his forehead, throwing daggers of Jesuitical logic at you. It was always an enormously challenging experience which doubled my blood pressure.

This time it was Adams who took the main stand. He had prepared a mini-lecture with a giant sketch pad, almost as big as himself, and he used a lecture baton to point out the reasons why Duesberg maintained in 1987, and still today, that HIV cannot cause AIDS. HIV is a retrovirus which, unlike the ordinary self-sufficient hand-grenade viruses that invade a cell and explode outwards, has to knit itself into its host cell in order to survive. It is identified when certain antibodies said to be specific to HIV are found in the bloodstream. Duesberg's case that HIV is a harmless hitch-hiker rested on the following key points:

- *There are very low levels of HIV in the body, which never rise, even in advanced AIDS.* When an ordinary virus causes disease, like viral pneumonia, the virus affecting a patient's lungs would actively infect over 70 per cent of lung cells and be readily seen in an electron micrograph. But the retrovirus HIV can hardly ever be found, even when AIDS patients who have died undergo an autopsy. HIV remains latent and inactive and at very low levels in those who test HIV positive with no symptoms of AIDS, and also in those who develop AIDS. There is not one report of a high virus level in blood from an AIDS patient. The virus can only be detected from 50 per cent of people with or without symptoms of AIDS. Even then, the virus cannot be found directly in blood taken from people with AIDS. It has to be activated using cell cultures, with the help of heroic laboratory techniques. This is done in the laboratory dish away from the body's immune responses and its natural protective reactions. In other words the conditions under which HIV is cultured are artificial and disconnected from the body's natural controlling responses to it.

• *There are too few infected cells in the body for HIV to cause disease.* HIV actively infects only 1 in 10,000 to 100,000 T (thymus) cells (these are cells crucial to the body's immune system, that protect against disease). Yet the body regenerates 5 per cent of T-cells in the two days it takes the virus to infect the cell. It is like an army with a continuing swell of reinforcements. Therefore, even if the virus killed every cell it infected, the body would regenerate them at a faster rate and the effect would be minimal.

• *The latency period, from infection with HIV to full-blown AIDS, does not make sense. In the early 1980s it was said to be five years, yet by the early 1990s latency was extended to 30 years.* If HIV were to be truly pathogenic (deadly), it would be expected to kill T-cells and cause AIDS when it first infects an organism and not years later. It would be required to reproduce itself in its host cell then burst out, killing the host cell and going on to infect hundreds of thousands of other healthy cells. But retroviruses like HIV cannot do this. Unlike our hand-grenade viruses that enter a cell and kill it, retroviruses do not typically kill cells because they cannot reproduce themselves without their host cell. They need to take up residence in their host cell and can only replicate themselves at the same rate as their host cell divides (mitosis).

- *There are cases of HIV infection with no AIDS.* According to figures from the US Centers for Disease Control, the number of estimated HIV positive people in the USA has remained at a steady 1.5 million ever since 1982 (more recently it is reported to have gone down to 750,000). Yet, Duesberg noted in his early papers, in any one year only 1 per cent of those (15,000) developed AIDS and only half of those (fewer than 0.5 per cent of all HIV positives) died. This meant that between 98 and 99 per cent of people who are estimated to be HIV positive in any year did not develop AIDS.

These were Duesberg's key arguments in 1987. They have not changed, and later he extended the list of inconsistencies to include the documented cases of AIDS with no trace of HIV infection.[1] Centers for Disease Control (CDC) data have subsequently shown that 10 per cent of cases diagnosed as AIDS have no sign of antibody to HIV. Of the 80–90 per cent of people with AIDS who do show antibody to HIV, in only 10 per cent can actual provirus (the integrated genetic material of the virus itself as opposed to antibodies to it) be found, most of which comprises defective (incomplete) viral particles, which cannot replicate.

Subsequent recent attempts have been made by David Ho and others[2] to show a massive viral activity of HIV. This 'viral load' they claim was detected through the use of PCR (polymerase chain reaction) for which Kary Mullis won a Nobel prize. But this work has been shown to be flawed by Kary Mullis himself, Peter Duesberg, working with his colleague Harvey Bialy, science editor of *Bio/Technology*,[3] Serge Lang, a mathematics professor at Yale University,[4] and Professor Mark Craddock of the School of Mathematics and Statistics, University of Sydney, Australia, who dismissed the mathematical model used. They maintain that what are being identified are non-infectious viral particles – in other words, particles that are incapable of going on to infect other cells. Their criticisms stem from the fact that the method used (PCR), which amplifies DNA and can find a needle in a haystack, can only tell you that genetic material is there, but cannot measure the quantity of virus.

Dissenting Voices: Why were they not Heard?

Having secured Channel 4's agreement to our proposal, within two weeks Adams, Verney-Elliott and the crew were off to film in New York and San Francisco. Jad, as director, had sent the rushes back after interviewing Duesberg in San Francisco. I remember walking from our office in Covent Garden into Soho one morning, to our film editor, Alan Ballard's cutting room. There we viewed Verney-Elliott's interview with Duesberg. Alan and I were rooted to our chairs. 'This is dynamite!' I said, as I heard Duesberg's clipped German accent. He spoke like a natural teacher. He made even the most complicated scientific principles understandable to a lay listener, mixing his explanations with liberal dashes of the kind of irony and humour that never failed to rile his opponents, helping to turn them from professional antagonists into personal enemies.

Adams and Verney-Elliott set about the painstaking process of piecing the film together, producing a series of rough cuts and then a near-final version for David Lloyd to see. The film reflected the views of several AIDS doubters. One of them was John Beldekas, an immunologist from Boston, who had two key points to make. The first concerned the anomalies he had discovered about the spread of HIV. He and his colleagues had conducted a survey of HIV prevalence in newborn babies in the state of Massachusetts. To his surprise he found that the level of infection, about 1.2 per cent, was the same in Boston's middle-class families as for the run-down inner city areas. This was reflected right across the state, indicating to him that HIV itself was not restricted to the then known risk groups – i.e. mainly intravenous drug users and homosexuals.

Beldekas concluded by saying, 'To my knowledge, even though there are many HIV positive babies in the state of Massachusetts, there really aren't many babies with AIDS. So there's a question right there. How can you have a high frequency of virus and not show a lot of frank AIDS cases?'[5] Beldekas was also concerned about the artificiality and the 'tremendous amount of unnatural laboratory steps' required to isolate a virus like HIV in an AIDS patient.

Basically what they do is take a lot of white blood cells which presumably are infected, put them in culture, put them in a test tube and bombard them with all types of chemicals, drugs, stimulators, that in some way change those white cells and coax out the virus. Now, as a person growing a virus, I could take a cell from your body, from your neck, and under the appropriate laboratory conditions, I could coax out a lot of viruses that you have been exposed to. Firstly, that doesn't mean you are a walking carrier that is shedding viruses and secondly it doesn't mean that you are potentially infectious. The carrying of these organisms we have been exposed to is called persistence – they persist within us and we can find them if we look with the right techniques.[6]

Even if the HIV virus is found, Duesberg chimes in:

It is dormant all the time. It never becomes active. It is dormant to begin with, it's dormant when [says the orthodoxy] you die from it. It's dormant when [says the orthodoxy] you suffer from it. There's no report in the literature describing the virus ever to be active in a patient. So it's always dormant. That is in fact one of the paradoxes of the viral hypothesis. There is no parasite that I know of among viruses, bacteria, fungus – anything – that is dormant while it is pathogenic. This one [they say] is! That's one of the major reasons why I don't believe that this virus is the cause of AIDS.[7]

Duesberg pointed to another glaring anomaly. 'The best evidence there is that the [HIV] virus is associated with AIDS patients is antibody to the virus, which is not the same as virus. At best it's an indirect test. In fact, it is almost an argument against the virus because typically, antibody to the virus means vaccination, protection.'[8] The film also allowed other scientists, doctors and journalists to express their disagreement with the virus/AIDS hypothesis, many of them frustrated because their grant applications for research into areas not dependent on an infectious viral cause for AIDS, were consistently turned down.

Dr Richard Ablin, for example, of the State University of New York was on record as saying that HIV was not the cause of AIDS but was simply 'a passenger on an already sinking ship'. Dr Ablin believed that damage to the immune system must come first and he had been looking for possible causes of this immune suppression. On film, he told reporter Verney-Elliott that he believed he had definitive evidence that an enzyme called transglutaminase, which was present both in semen and in the clotting factor concentrates like Factor VIII, taken by haemophiliacs, contributed to immune suppression. If transglutaminase in semen could cause problems to the immune system, asked Verney-Elliott, why aren't more women getting AIDS-like symptoms? 'The problem here,' Ablin replied, 'is that the lining of the rectum is much thinner than the lining of the vagina and so one could envision that the type of trauma that might be associated with anal intercourse would be much more severe than that which could occur in the vagina.'[9]

Another view came from New York doctor Stephen Caiazza. He believed AIDS was due to syphilis being poorly treated with the wrong kind of penicillin, which did not kill off all the organisms causing the disease. Some remained in the central nervous system. He also maintained that many cases of syphilis have never been diagnosed and therefore never been correctly eradicated, spreading the disease further in the susceptible gay population.

The programme also included an interview with Chuck Ortleb, editor of the gay weekly paper, *New York Native*. He had always strongly questioned the theory that HIV causes AIDS, and mounted a number of campaigns to attract public attention to alternative theories. He supported the work of Boston scientist Jane Teas, who, together with John Beldekas, had worked on the theory that AIDS could be a human result of African swine fever virus infection. There had been reports in the scientific literature of a number of AIDS patients who appeared to be infected with this virus. They found it impossible to get any support for their work.

Why did Ortleb doubt HIV when all the leading laboratories and scientists did not? 'If you started interviewing all of the scientists in those laboratories', he said, 'you'd find there was a lot of doubt out there. They're afraid to speak up because they'll be punished. They will lose their grants and they will lose their jobs. AIDS science is really a religion, and if you dare challenge authority you lose your livelihood. That's the way science works.'[10] This was indeed to be the case for Dr Ablin, whose laboratory was closed down, and for Peter Duesberg himself, who was to arouse the wrath of the scientific establishment and suffer accordingly.

The programme also looked at the financial interests surrounding the AIDS business. At the Chiron Corporation in California, work was proceeding in the search for a vaccine against HIV. Dr Dino Dina told us that from start of development to final approval a vaccine could cost $20 to $30 million to develop.

The sale of HIV test kits had become a source of immense revenue. Each time a drop of blood was tested, it meant 43 pence for the company producing the kit. Many scientists researching into the AIDS virus themselves had companies selling test kits and owned millions of dollars in company shares. AIDS for these individuals was a very profitable business. 'What we should really find out is what the true cause of AIDS is,' concluded Duesberg:

and in order to do this we have to work with the patient or go back to the clinic or back on to the streets or in the bathhouses – or study those who are at risk. The haemophiliacs or the high risk promiscuous male homosexuals and intravenous drug users, and see what in fact AIDS is. AIDS is not a disease entity. AIDS is a whole bag of old diseases under a new name.[11]

We did find Duesberg compelling, both in his discourse and personality. At the very least, we felt, his arguments deserved serious attention.

AIDS: The Unheard Voices was transmitted in Channel 4's *Dispatches* strand on Tuesday, 8 September 1987. We thought our film would change the world, but it fell into a pool of professional silence. Not a single medical journal or medical correspondent deigned to put a toe in the water on the subject. The general press, on the other hand, was far more favourably disposed towards a questioning of scientific orthodoxy. Liz Cowley in the *Daily Mail*, described the programme as 'astonishing'. 'Do they [doctors] know', she wrote, 'on what scale some scientists are now questioning the theory that HIV causes AIDS?'[12] The *Independent* called the programme 'important and accessible'. Christopher Tookey of the *Sunday Telegraph* wrote:

The outstanding documentary of this and many weeks turned out to be the second in Channel 4's new journalistic series Dispatches. *This argued with surprisingly strong evidence that AIDS is not caused by HIV. If the programme's thesis is true then it's both bad and good news. The bad news is that much of the world's AIDS research is being wasted on finding a vaccine for the wrong virus. The good news is that a lot of people who now think they may be going to die of AIDS are not, in fact, going to do anything of the kind. ... The makers of this highly controversial documentary must have agonized for many hours about whether to make it or not. It will undoubtedly have depressed many who are working in the field flat out on finding a cure for HIV. On the other hand, of course, the programme's thesis may be right. It was certainly well argued, and can only do good if it helps to stop what may have been a tragic misdirection of resources.*[13]

Our greatest satisfaction came after David Lloyd decided to submit our film for the Royal Television Society (RTS) journalism awards. After a good dinner and large brandy as guests of Liz Forgan on the Channel 4 table at the Grosvenor House awards ceremony, the prize winners were announced by Paul Fox. And we won! Jad Adams, Michael Verney-Elliott and I won the RTS's award for international journalism and that night became the first independents ever to win an RTS award. After dealing with our elation and encouraged by the award from our peers we started building up our archive for the next programme. It was during this period that Adams decided to write his book. He wrote much of it in our office at the desk next to mine.

AIDS: The HIV Myth was published by Macmillan in 1989. When it came out it received high praise in the national press and from both the *Lancet* and *Nature*. The *Lancet* (which was later to become distinctly hostile on this issue) called it a 'spirited attack on received wisdom. ... Does an excellent job of summarizing doubts about AIDS/ HIV.'[14] In *Nature*, virologist Professor Beverly Griffin wrote:

Meticulously researched. ... Named scientists are the butt of Adams' invective as he draws attention to their abandonment of the scientific approach, acquisition of vested interests in the virus they champion and use of steam-roller tactics to silence any opposition. . . . Adams has written a highly provocative but important book on a huge medical problem. It deserves to be read.[15]

But Duncan Campbell thought differently. Enraged by the fact that Adams described AIDS as a 'behavioural disease', which Campbell considered 'offensive to AIDS sufferers', he poured out a stream of invective in a review in the *New Scientist*, 'His [Adams's] reporting is staggeringly inaccurate, scientifically inept, and continually blighted by the misinterpretation or distortion of the minimal scientific sources that he has consulted. He has constructed his book in such remarkable ignorance of so much widely available research and information on AIDS and immunology that it is very hard to believe that his ignorance is not deliberate.'[16]

When an invitation arrived to debate his book with Duncan Campbell at a meeting at the London School of Economics (LSE), Adams had no idea what was in store for him. Campbell was a member of a group called Campaign Against Health Fraud, also known as Quackbusters, some of whose members appeared to be linked with the pharmaceutical industry. Campbell had been building up steam about Duesberg's arguments. In the event, the viciousness of Campbell's attack on Adams at the LSE took him completely unawares. Adams had been expecting a scientific debate on the evidence but instead walked into a personal attack.

Martin Walker, in his book *Dirty Medicine*, describes the following scene.

For Jad Adams, Campbell had nothing but seething contempt. He attacked the book, not on the grounds that the arguments could be wrong and might be open to debate, but on the grounds that it had been badly written by a stupid person. [Campbell said] 'Nothing in this book makes any sense. It is, to be blunt, unmitigated clap-trap from beginning to end. Every key scientific statement in it is wrong, and provably wrong, and discoverably wrong. It's sloppy. It's self-contradictory.'[17]

Campbell's efforts have been consistent in one respect: he seldom offered any scientific arguments to back up his position. He simply acted like a Nintendo exterminator. He could not possibly have known of Duesberg's background and renown among his peers in the field of retrovirology and he certainly could not have read any of his papers when he declared, 'What we have here in Duesberg, is a mad ego-maniac. Nothing in this book is scientific. Duesberg is capable of writing the most appalling crap.' And later, 'There are people getting on with the job (dealing with AIDS) and there are, to be frank, idiots like Duesberg, getting in the way, with no science to back them up.'[18]

Campbell's vituperation knew no bounds. Even Macmillan, Jad Adams's publishers, were flailed. 'I hope they'll undertake to us [*sic*], that if they find the facts to be wrong, as the scientists and doctors will tell them that they are, that the book will be withdrawn from sale, before it can do further harm, by putting out erroneous information.'[19] Campbell's attack was continued in the pages of the *New Scientist*. Macmillan's editorial director, Adam Sisman, jumped to Adams's defence in a letter to the *New Scientist* calling Campbell's review of Adams's book 'wild and unpleasant'. He said, 'I want to refute some of your more hysterical criticisms of Macmillan as the publishers of the book.'[20] Far from being intimidated, Macmillan proceeded to commission another book from Adams.

Criticism of Adams's book also came from the medical establishment. Dr Anthony Pinching wrote, 'The book reads like a manifesto of the Flat Earth Society.'[21] The attempt to suppress any view about AIDS that differed from the orthodoxy was in full swing. Both the medical establishment and much of the media were obviously unsympathetic to John Stuart Mill's famous plea for tolerance of other people's ideas:

If all mankind minus one, were of one opinion and only one person were of the contrary opinion, mankind would be no more justified in silencing that one person, than he if he had the power, would be justified in silencing mankind. . . . We can never be sure that the opinion we are endeavouring to stifle is a false opinion; and if we were sure, stifling it would be an evil still.[22]

Chapter 3

Life in Backrooms and Bathhouses

The Risk/AIDS Hypothesis

When it became clear that gays weren't going away, a commercialized, consumerist version of sexuality was conceded to us, a sexuality all the more frantic for being emptied of deep emotion. This fuelled a machine without oil, which could only burn itself out until it seized up completely.

(Ian Young, *The Stonewall Experiment*, 1995)

It was young gay men who were first identified in 1981 as having GRID (gay related immune deficiency) which was later called AIDS. Early suggestions were that AIDS was linked with a gay lifestyle. This naturally offended the gay community. However, as the years went by the predominant group of people with AIDS were still drawn from the gay community, albeit that small percentage who were very promiscuous and abused drugs to enhance their sexual activity. So might the promiscuous gay lifestyle hypothesis have some truth in it? It is important to document here how gay men themselves describe their awareness of the health risks involved for those who chose the gay 'fast lane'. Michael Callen was an enormously attractive man. He was slim and sensuous with a look that positively exuded sex appeal. He was the embodiment of the new 'gay' man. In his slow laconic drawl, he expressed himself with immense fluency, a quality he used to great advantage as a public speaker. He was also a gifted singer and cabaret performer.

I first met him on the shoot for our documentary *The AIDS Catch*. We knew that he did not believe HIV was the cause of AIDS and were keen to interview him. He agreed to fly to Boston for our interview while he was on tour with his cabaret group. As he devoured the hotel's room service food late that night, he told me of those early days of gay liberation at Harvard when sex became the most important thing in his life. 'By the time I was 23,' he said, 'I had had 2000 partners.' 'I was very, very active in the sexual revolution of the late 1970s and 1980s. I have a long distinguished list of sexually transmitted infections and I assumed that at the same time I was getting syphilis, gonorrhoea and non-specific urethritis, hepatitis, CMV [cytomegalovirus] and EBV [Epstein–Barr virus], that I also picked up HIV.'[1]

Callen thought he had been HIV positive since 1983, before testing came in, and was already famous for his book *Surviving AIDS*.[2] He was also well-known for openly questioning HIV as the cause of AIDS and for an article he wrote with Richard Berkowitz in the *New York Native* in 1982 called 'We know who we are'. The article was written before HIV was announced to be the cause of AIDS and before the virus/AIDS hypothesis swamped any good old-fashioned, on-the-ground risk factor analysis. In retrospect, it was a truly prophetic piece of writing.

'Can researchers really comprehend the dynamics of urban gay male promiscuity?' he wrote. 'The commercialization of promiscuity and the explosion of establishments such as bathhouses, bookstores, and backrooms is unique in western history.' 'Do the gay communities of New York, San Francisco, and Los Angeles realize that promiscuity has become such a narcotic for some that we know of men who have been diagnosed with AIDS and Kaposi's sarcoma and who, even in the face of imminent death, are at this moment "moderating" their sexual habits at the baths and backrooms?'

We believe that it is the accumulation of risk through leading a promiscuous gay urban lifestyle which has led to the breakdown of the immune responses that we are seeing now. Most published medical reports indicate that continued re-exposure and reinfection with common viruses (most notably cytomegalovirus), in conjunction with other common venereal infections and perhaps other factors, have led to the present health crisis among urban gay promiscuous men. 'Continued re-exposure and rein-fection with common infections' means bathhouse/backroom sexual activity.[3]

Although the famous article lingers mainly on the risk of re-exposure and reinfection, Callen and Berkowitz also mention other risk factors that depress the immune system, like intravenous and other drug usage, stress and diet.

An important influence on Callen had been his doctor, Joseph Sonnabend, a respected New York physician and editor of the pioneering AIDS dissident magazine *AIDS Research*. He had treated many AIDS patients in his practice in central Manhattan and believed that AIDS was caused by a multiplicity of different factors acting together. Sonnabend had observed that the social behaviour of certain homosexual men was exposing them to successive sexually transmitted infections from common microorganisms that were known to have had immune suppressive components. Callen recognized the possible lifestyle factors associated with AIDS and, as a leader in the gay community, began to disseminate information about the risk/AIDS hypothesis. 'It suggested to me there were multiple targets against which to direct therapy. So immediately it had practical significance to me. If AIDS was caused by a variety of factors acting all at once, then if I could knock out any one of them like dominoes I could maybe stop the chain of events that was making me sick.'[4]

Callen's article in the *New York Native* caused a furore among the gay community. Callen was 'roasted alive' by many of his peers who felt that when Reagan was elected, a new conservatism came into being, and any suggestion that lifestyle played a role in making people sick 'would play into the new right tendency to say, they brought it on themselves, let them die.'[5]

Callen told me that when HIV came on the map, many gay leaders, though largely persuaded of the multifactorial risk hypothesis (repeated reinfections and a fast-track drug-associated lifestyle) took a conscious decision, for political reasons, to support the 'no blame' virus/AIDS hypothesis. But Callen and Berkowitz didn't back down. 'My view', said Callen, 'was that you had to tell the truth to guys, because if you didn't tell them the truth bluntly in language they could understand, they would kill themselves, and I felt there was an ethical imperative to speak from my own experience.'[6] The Callen and Berkowitz article led to the closure of 14 bathhouses in San Francisco and many others across America. Callen's condition began to deteriorate in 1993. He died a year later.

So What Went On in Backrooms and Bathhouses?

In some of New York and San Francisco's bathhouses, as you walked in a tray was offered with a range of antibiotic cocktails to take as an aperitif, supposedly to help protect against the soup of sexually transmissible infections waiting inside. Then onwards and inwards. Dennis Altman in his book *Homosexual Oppression and Liberation* describes them:

These resemble nothing so much as giant steaming whorehouses in which everyone is a customer; clad only in white towels men prowl the hallways, groping each other in furtive search for instant sex, making it in small dark cubicles on low, hard, come-stained beds. Disgusting? – yes, perhaps. Yet lasting friendships are quite commonly begun in bathhouses and to this extent the whorehouse analogy is not fully accurate. It is a feature of male homosexual life that sex usually precedes intimacy to a much greater extent than among heterosexuals.[7]

Backrooms were to be found in most capital cities across America and Europe. They were the special areas in popular gay bars where patrons could indulge in wild promiscuous sex frequently involving sado-masochism, fisting and all the most excessive forms of gay sex. The sexual activity was of such intensity that drugs were needed to fuel it. At the height of bathhouse and backroom activity, more than 70 different chemical stimulants or depressants were commonly used by the dedicated 'fast tracker'. Backrooms usually had very low lighting or were indeed pitch dark to facilitate anonymity. David Black in his *Rolling Stone* article 'The Plague Years' writes, 'The gay baths and backrooms, with their poor hygiene, mimicked the unhealthy conditions of equatorial Africa. . . . They were, in a way no one previously suspected, a sexual Third World.'[8]

Drugs and Disco Devotees

Before the visit to the backroom or bathhouse often came the disco where other dangers lay. When we interviewed John Lauritsen for *The AIDS Catch* he expressed his concern about repeated sexually transmitted infections and their treatment with broad spectrum antibiotics, which were immune-suppressant, and went on to describe visits to discotheques and leather clubs:

They would take drugs, not just a few drugs, not innocuous drugs, but they might take six different drugs in the course of an evening. And we don't really know the consequences of these drugs. But they would include poppers which are nitrite inhalants, MDA [methylenedioxyamphetamine] which is a designer drug, even Ecstasy and Special K which are other designer drugs. And they would include ethyl chloride, a deadly substance which is inhaled. It would also include cocaine and heroin and marijuana and alcohol. And if people took half a dozen of these things in the course of an evening, who knows what the interaction effects are? Who knows what the long-term effects of any one of them is separately?[9]

In 1983, Lauritsen interviewed Artie Felson, a founder of People with AIDS, New York and a member (as Lauritsen was) of the New York Safer Sex Committee. 'He [Felson] told me,' writes Lauritsen:

that he had interviewed between 300 and 400 gay men with 'AIDS', and had interrogated each of them with regard to sex and drug use. Though none of his respondents were virgins, some of them had not been especially 'promiscuous'. However, they were all drug users. Felson said he had heard stories of drug abuse that would make the hair stand on end. And, without a single exception, they had all used poppers. My conversations with Felson took place before the 'AIDS/virus' hypothesis had become obligatory Truth, so we were still free to bandy about ideas as to what 'AIDS' was and what caused it. Felson adamantly maintained that he himself had become sick as a consequence of drug abuse, and that 'AIDS' itself represented drug injuries to the body.[10]

In his novel *Faggots*, Larry Kramer lists 76 favourite drugs of the Fire Island gay scene, among them MDA, MDMA (Ecstacy), YHC, PCP (angel dust) STP, DMT, LDK, WDW, mescaline, strychnine and mantanuska thunderfuck. He provides a glimpse into drug usage at a Manhattan gay disco: "'I'm trying something new," Tarsh yelled. . . . It's called Super K, it's from England, it's a pre-op sedative used for children, it's a powder to snort, a cross between coke and valium and it's fabulous!'[11]

Duesberg has for many years stressed that intravenous drug use and long-term exposure to recreational drugs is what causes the initial breakdown of the immune system, which then allows opportunistic infections to take over the undefended body. He is particularly concerned about the effects of these drugs on sleeping and eating patterns. What he describes as a life of 'Uppers and downers – not sleeping, not eating'. Several years of that, he says, and you'll die young.

By the late 1970s the gay fast-track lifestyle and disco-drugs scene had spread to most European capitals. Before a man went on the town he needed a lift to get out of the house, then at the disco he would try something else at the bar, then on the dance floor he might sniff the poppers bottle slung around his neck, and then maybe some more during sex that night. And this could go on every night of the week. Topping the popularity list were poppers and a variety of Ecstasy whose ingredients were claimed to include heroin. No one seemed to think poppers could be damaging. Most men frequenting these fast-track gay clubs thought it was just like taking a cup of tea. None of the major AIDS organizations properly warned about the dangers of drugs. Drugs were portrayed as risky only in that they might affect 'judgement' and facilitate a lapse into 'unsafe sex'.

'Poppers', said John Lauritsen, 'which cause genes to mutate, which cause severe anaemia, which can kill through heart attacks, which suppress the immune system – are depicted as bad only if they cause someone to forget about condoms.'[12] Instead of advising readers of the dangers of these recreational drugs, gay magazines carried advertisements for them and in editorial features even provided advice on how to store them in the fridge.[13] Although none of the 'official' AIDS organizations has taken a strong stand against drugs in the gay scene, one group, Positively Healthy, had steadily stood its ground. Its co-founder, Cass Mann, had consistently warned about the links between drug toxicity and AIDS. He was particularly concerned about the worrying evidence linking poppers with Kaposi's sarcoma, the skin lesions affecting many gay men with AIDS.[14]

What is it that drove some gay men on to a level of promiscuity that required one sexual adventure after another? Two well-known writers on gay sexuality, Camille Paglia and David Black have their own views. Paglia sees gay men as guardians of the masculine impulse, 'To have anonymous sex in a dark alleyway is to pay homage to the dream of male freedom. The unknown stranger is a wandering pagan god. The altar, as in prehistory, is anywhere you kneel.'[15] David Black describes the compulsive sexuality of some men as:

The erotic equivalent of eating salted peanuts. Once you've put sex at the centre of your identity whether you say, 'I am a gay man' or 'I am a straight stud' you need a constant series of sexual adventures, each one upping the ante of the others, in order to nourish your sense of self. What happens when that need slams up against your instinct for survival?[16]

The post-Vietnam surge in drug taking coincided with the gay liberation movement of the 1960s and 1970s. The results, in terms of promiscuity among some, were explosive. Emerging gays needing to determine their sexual identity required more and more sexual contacts and these became impossible without drug assisted sex.

In his 1992 paper 'The role of drugs in the origin of AIDS',[17] Peter Duesberg points out that the appearance of AIDS in America coincided with a massive escalation in the consumption of recreational drugs that started in the 1960s and 1970s. He quotes the Bureau of Justice statistics reports that the number of drug arrests in the USA rose from 450,000 in 1980 to 1.4 million in 1989; that the Drug Enforcement Administration confiscated about 9000 kilograms of cocaine in 1980 compared with 100,000 kilograms in 1990; that the National Institute on Drug Abuse reported that in 1979–80 over five million people used nitrite inhalants in the USA at least once a week. In his summary Duesberg writes, 'Epidemiologically, both epidemics (drugs and AIDS) derive about 80 per cent of their victims from the same groups of 20–44 year-olds, of which 90 per cent are males. In the USA, 32 per cent of these are intravenous drug users and their children, about 60 per cent are male homosexual.' He then goes on to explain his view that the American AIDS epidemic is a subset of the drugs epidemic. For example, when an HIV negative drug addict gets pneumonia, TB or dementia, it is described as such, but when an HIV positive drug addict suffers from the same conditions he is diagnosed as having AIDS. 'If you've got dementia plus HIV,' says Duesberg, 'you're told you've got AIDS. But if you've got dementia, period, you're just stupid!' But the darker side to this story is that any HIV positive drug addict with AIDS-associated conditions were prescribed AZT with all its associated toxicity. These patients have not survived.

In the three years between 1984 and 1987, deaths among intra-venous drug users in New York, whether diagnosed with AIDS or whether suffering from non-AIDS pneumonia and septicaemia, increased at exactly the same rate. This led the US Centers for Disease Control to acknowledge, 'We cannot discern, however, to what extent the upward trend in death rates for drug abuse reflects trends in illicit drug use independent of the HIV epidemic.' Duesberg's views on the link between drugs and AIDS is supported in a study by Dr Maurizio Lucà Moretti. He studied 508 former intravenous drug users (190 HIV positive) in a rehabilitation centre in Italy. All of them had malnutrition during the period of their addiction. He found that the longer the men had taken drugs, and the higher the dose, the more likely they were to suffer immune impairment and the more likely they were to be HIV positive. 'This leads to the conclusion,' writes Moretti, 'that the degree of insults to the immune system is directly correlated to HIV seroconversion.' When the drugs were withdrawn and the men received adequate nutri-tion and avoided sexually-transmitted diseases, none of the HIV positive subjects showed any symptoms of AIDS or AIDS related diseases.[18]

Young drug addicts had been dying on the streets of London and New York (with AIDS-like symptoms) years before AIDS ever appeared. Emeritus Professor of Public Health at Glasgow University, Gordon Stewart, made a study of drug addiction in New York City in the 1960s.

They were getting all sorts of opportunistic infections, probably passed on by needles. Eighty five to ninety per cent of them had evidence of hepatitis. They were often extremely emaciated, suffering from wasting diseases, various weird bloodborne infections with skin bacteria, Candida and Cryptococci, which would not ordinarily be regarded as pathogenic in their own right. . . . We didn't find Kaposi's sarcoma and we didn't find Pneumocystis (carinii pneumonia or PCP) but, then, we weren't looking for it.[19]

Journalist Darrell Yates Rist writes of New York: 'Someone reports the death of a junkie, the body is taken away and put down as an overdose. No one is going to do an open lung smear on that person to find out if they really died of pneumocystis.' Gordon Stewart had once told me that death certificates for drug addicts are often written out by psychiatrists in drug addiction units who are not always interested in the finer clinical details of the cause of death. I telephoned London's Maudsley Hospital and spoke to a consultant in its drug unit. What were the most common causes of death? Pneumonia, septicaemia (infection of the blood) and pericarditis (inflammation of the heart lining), I was told. These are all AIDS related conditions, did he not think AIDS could be a manifestation of drug abuse regardless of HIV? 'Certainly not,' he said.

The trouble is that commitment to HIV as the sole cause of AIDS has left important areas like these completely unresearched. Duesberg has repeatedly applied for funding for research into the drug/AIDS hypothesis both from the NIH and from private sources and has received one rejection after another. None of the investigations into drug use and abuse among AIDS patients is satisfactory. Voluntary reporting in interviews and questionnaires can hardly be relied upon in a climate where drugs are illegal and homosexuality itself unacceptable to the majority of the population.

In 1985 David Black quoted Virginia Apuzzo, former executive director of the National Gay Task Force, on this subject:

Homosexuality is still a felony in twenty-three states. How the hell do they expect us to answer questions like what drugs do we use and what do we do sexually? Where is this information going? Into what computer bank?

Do you want a list of 10 million sick men who are also homosexual? I resisted the paranoia, but instinctive things go off in a crisis that make you remember you are not dealing with friendly institutions. It's a little like asking blacks in 1964 to trust labour unions that came to their assistance. Thank you very much. Next![20]

Whatever the explanation for the promiscuity of some gays and their bathhouse habits and drug abuse, it seems closely linked with Michael Callen's unflinching admission that the very same lifestyle was the cause of his illness:

It became impossible for me to pretend that the disease history was irrelevant to the fact that I was sick. It was sort of emotionally attractive to believe that it had nothing to do with any choices I had made, that it was just bad luck – I'd accidentally slept with the wrong person. But, once I was presented with a non-moralistic, calm, medical presentation of a multi-factorial mechanism which might account for my illness I was never quite able to believe again that a disease of this complexity was ever going to have a single, simple cause.[21]

Chapter 4

Hunting the Human Retrovirus

The Feud Begins:
Discord among the Kings of Virology

Berlin World AIDS Conference, 1993

H e walked into the conference hall like a Hollywood film star at a premier, with a huge smile and three bodyguards. But he wasn't a film star, he was virologist Robert Gallo, the man who claimed to have discovered HIV, by now assumed to be the cause of AIDS. As he made his way to his seat in the press auditorium, few journalists cared to remember that he had admitted accidentally misappropriating Luc Montagnier's AIDS virus isolate, calling it his own, and few journalists had noticed that in that very month Gallo had been found guilty of scientific misconduct by his peers.

This verdict of misconduct was reached by the Department of Health and Human Services' Office of Research Integrity (ORI). It concluded that Gallo and his colleague Mikulas Popovic had made false statements in published science papers. Gallo was accused of having intentionally misled colleagues to gain credit for himself and diminish credit due to his French competitors. The report also said that his false statement had 'impeded potential AIDS research progress' by diverting scientists from potentially fruitful work with the French researchers. Later, the Department of Health and Human Services' appeals board looked into Popovic's case first and decided on new criteria for the definition of scientific misconduct. 'Intent to deceive' had to be proved. The board cleared Popovic, saying it had found 'no palpable wrongdoing'.[1] On this narrow interpretation by a board of lawyers not scientists, the ORI decided it had to drop Gallo's case and charges of misconduct were withdrawn. The goal posts had been moved yet again to protect the orthodoxy (see Chapter 11).

Many journalists at the conference may also not have known that in the preceding year several members of Gallo's laboratory team had been investigated for various malpractices, including the removal of government financed viral isolates, reagents and other materials out of the laboratory for use in their own private biotechnology companies. Today, however, Gallo was the star of the show, at the 1993 Berlin World AIDS Conference, and the show must go on.

Round the corner in central Berlin, fellow retrovirologist Peter Duesberg, once Gallo's friend but now considered by Gallo to be his arch enemy, was having coffee with a group of AIDS dissidents. Duesberg had not been invited to the conference and within hours he was on the plane back to his laboratories at Berkeley, California. The feud between these two men began soon after the famous press conference in 1984, when US Health Secretary Margaret Heckler, with Gallo by her side, announced, 'The probable cause of AIDS has been found.' Duesberg had worked on retroviruses with Gallo at the NIH, and had been the first scientist to map the genetic sequence of a retrovirus. So when the official announcement was made that the retrovirus HIV could cause AIDS, he was astonished. 'It can't do it,' he said to himself. 'HIV just can't kill all those cells. There isn't a mechanism for it.'

As the HIV bandwagon began to roll, Duesberg began to write. His first paper, critical of the HIV/AIDS hypothesis in *Cancer Research*[2] had attracted a fair amount of attention among his peers and made Gallo his enemy. Strange, because Gallo had once described Duesberg as the 'guy who knows more about retroviruses than anyone else in the world.' At a scientific conference in Germany in 1985, he introduced Duesberg as 'brilliant and original, a scientist of extraordinary energy, unusual honesty, with an enormous sense of humour, and a rare critical sense which often makes us look twice, then a third time, at a conclusion many of us believed to be foregone'.[3]

But soon he would be insinuating that Duesberg was not only wrong but mad, and hung around with unsavoury characters 'in leather jackets'. As far back as 1988, Gallo described Duesberg's ideas as 'dangerous nonsense'. 'He has now indicated to people that they can go out and fuck around and get infected by this virus and not worry. That's the part where I am mad at Peter.'[4] For pointing out some uncomfortable truths to the scientific community Duesberg, once 'scientist of the year' three years running, academician of the US National Academy of Sciences and holder of an 'outstanding investigator's grant' from the US government, would soon find himself defrocked, defunded, shunned by his peers and even prevented from teaching postgraduate students.

How can the Whole World have Got it so Wrong about AIDS?

It is inconceivable, you will be saying, that in something as serious as AIDS, the whole of the scientific establishment, and indeed everyone else can have got it so wrong. If there is genuine doubt about HIV as the cause of AIDS, why are we not hearing the dissenting voices? Where is the debate? There are several reasons why those who put forward cogent scientific arguments against the virus/AIDS hypothesis are not heard. The censorship that exists in the peer review process operated by the leading scientific journals protects current orthodox views and prevents the airing of controversial arguments. Medical and science journalists tend to support a prevailing scientific orthodoxy. To challenge it could undermine public confidence in the scientific establishment. The doctor is still God, and government health policies dictated by doctors and scientists should not be questioned.

Then there is the inevitable desire to protect the immense sums of money involved in ten-year HIV-based research grants and patents for the various test kits and antiviral drugs. The story of AIDS is also special because this is the first time in the history of medicine that so much money has been thrown into one particular disease. With $40,000 million spent in 14 years in the USA, it is the biggest industry next to the defence department. This money was fuelled by the plague terror tactics used by well-established organizations like the US Centers for Disease Control and its offshoot, the Epidemic Intelligence

Service (EIS), whose members are strategically placed in positions of power and influence in the media.

There is yet another more complex reason for the support of an infectious agent as the cause of AIDS. In the West, those affected by the syndrome are 90 per cent male, of whom over 50 per cent are homosexual habitual drug users – both intravenous and recreational. During the 1980s, the gay community had a powerful lobbying voice with governments that were anxious to be seen to be 'politically correct'. An infectious cause for AIDS was more expedient for the gay community. It allowed gay men to feel that there was an external cause for their affliction, one that could also threaten the heterosexual community. It gave gay activist groups a *raison d'être*. Through their own experience, they could offer advice to heterosexuals about so-called 'safer sex'.

Once HIV was accepted as the cause of AIDS by the majority of gay men, a certain sense of relief entered their lives. They had seen many of their lovers and closest friends waste away before their eyes. Now they could grieve for them, knowing that HIV, this strange, novel virus, said to have come from Africa, had caused the death of their loved one, perhaps after only one 'unlucky' sexual encounter. Nothing to do with the fact that the friend or loved one had probably been sniffing nitrites (poppers) on the dance floor; or taking any one of fifty different 'recreational' chemical drugs night after night for years; might have had hundreds of sexual partners in a year; might have stopped eating and sleeping properly; and might have been taking antibiotics all year round for recurrent syphilis, gonorrhoea and hepatitis. No, the friend or loved one had definitely died of HIV. Anyone challenging the accepted cause of death was deeply resented, and quickly labelled homophobic. That was sacrilege. A resigned and sinister death worship began to creep into the AIDS-stricken communities.

How Ever Did HIV Take Off in the First Place?

To understand how HIV ever came to be adopted as the cause of AIDS, it is not enough simply to run through the well-rehearsed reasons advanced by the orthodoxy and then to list the points of disagreement offered by the scientists who challenge the established view. This is a far more interesting story. The story has to be told in context, carrying along with it the political and social climate surrounding the emergence of AIDS, and in particular the prevailing microclimates circling around the great virology laboratories of the times. The story focuses on three men:

- The dapper, quick tempered Robert Gallo and his circle of colleagues, known as the Bob Club, firmly ensconced in the glass and concrete laboratories of the National Cancer Institute, part of the NIH in Bethesda, Maryland;

- Luc Montagnier, the chubby, round-faced, rather diffident French scientist and his team at the Pasteur Institute in Paris who first isolated LAV/HIV; and

- Peter Duesberg, the gadfly in the ointment. Trim and athletic, steel-rimmed specs, thick mane of crinkly silver hair, the brilliant German molecular biologist with, they say, the best 'lab hands' in the business. Based in the Stanley Laboratory under the Berkeley campus fir trees in balmy California, Duesberg was the inspiration behind the setting up of the Group for the Scientific Reappraisal of HIV, comprising more than 350 scientists and health professionals who challenge the virus/AIDS hypothesis.

In a nutshell, Gallo became convinced that HIV is the cause of AIDS and that it is sufficient in itself to cause disease and death. In 1988, he told Anthony Liversidge in an interview for *Spin Magazine* that 'HIV killed like a truck' and that talk of co-factors is 'cock and horseshit ... baloney'.[5] He also said, in another interview, 'HIV would cause AIDS in Clark Kent [Superman] given the right dose and the right strain of the virus ... alone and of itself. No doubt in my mind.'[6]

Montagnier was never quite so sure HIV could cause AIDS all on its own. In the very early days he was not sure if HIV was doing anything at all. As far back as 1983 at the Cold Spring Harbor conference on human retroviruses, after describing his work on LAV – lymphadenopathy associated virus (later renamed HIV) – while emphasizing that LAV *might* cause the lymph node abnormalities in AIDS patients, he said

33

'many other retroviruses ... might be causing AIDS.' Seven years later he told us, 'At first, we thought we had the best candidate for this virus to be the cause of AIDS. But after a while, even from the beginning actually, we thought for the activation of the virus in cells we need some co-factors.' Montagnier believed that something else was needed – a co-factor or co-factors – in order to make HIV pathogenic (harmful). 'So I would agree that HIV by itself, or some strains of HIV are not sufficient to cause AIDS.'[7]

Duesberg believes HIV is not the cause of AIDS and that HIV is not biochemically active. It is simply a passenger, hitch-hiking retrovirus that lives with us and is chronically dormant. It is barely detectable and consistently latent even in people with AIDS. He maintains that HIV and retroviruses in general, unlike ordinary viruses, do not kill cells. Indeed, it was for this reason that for ten years, retroviruses were wrongly suspected of causing cancer – a disease of uncontrolled cell growth. Paradoxically, this same type of virus was now blamed for causing AIDS, a disease where cells apparently disappear.

Retroviruses knit themselves into the DNA of their host cell and need to live with it. Anyone testing positive for HIV is demonstrating that the body's own immune system has done a good job by producing antibodies and neutralizing the invader. Duesberg dismisses the co-factor theories by saying that introducing co-factors to bolster up a theory that is foundering is the sign of a bankrupt hypothesis. Or, as he put it to us, 'It's the beginning of the retreat from Moscow!'

In a 1994 interview for *Reappraising AIDS,* the journal produced by the Group for the Scientific Reappraisal of HIV Duesberg says:

In ten years of the most unprecedented research effort we have no evidence that HIV is causing AIDS. The contrary is true. We have one million Americans who are HIV positive and are healthy, eight million Africans are HIV positive for eight years and are healthy, and half a million Europeans are healthy. [Some] 150 chimpanzees inoculated with HIV don't get AIDS and have these antibodies. How come no doctor ever in ten years picked up AIDS from a patient when they have treated them and we have no vaccine? How come 15,000 haemophiliacs live for ten years with HIV and don't die from it – instead their median lifespan doubles?[8]

Duesberg and Gallo had been colleagues, but gradually they began to fall out in a big way. The duel between them is well known to those close to them. Duesberg's stories about Gallo are always accompanied by a generous helping of his wicked sense of humour. Perhaps the best documented account of their growing animosity is to be found in Gallo's section on Duesberg in his book *Virus Hunting*[9] and Duesberg's critique of the latter, 'On Virus Hunting' in the *New York Native*.[10] Gallo says, 'One can only point out that Duesberg is a chemist, a molecular virologist. No physician, no epidemiologist, no health worker from any part of the world to my knowledge would agree with this [his] view.' Duesberg replies, 'I wonder whether MD Gallo might not have been better cast using his medical training to treat AIDS patients than trying to resolve the "molecular virology" of HIV and the "chemistry" of AIDS.' Duesberg accuses Gallo of being so politically correct that he 'does not want to offend American homosexuals or central Africans and their microbes by assuring all of us that sexual transmission man to woman ... is probably the most common pathway to infection in the world and not man to man by sex, as we in the US tend to think. That however,' continues Duesberg, 'leaves open the question as to why women represent less than 10 per cent of all AIDS cases in the US.' Gallo says, 'Duesberg's rush to the media has its dangerous side.' To which Duesberg replies, 'But Gallo, the father of science by press release, fails to explain why it is "dangerous" for me, Montagnier, and others who question a hypothesis that in seven years of fierce research and annual investments that currently amount to 3×10^{10} dollars has yet to stop or contain AIDS, or even predict its spread.'

Although this sparring is entertaining, the key scientific differences of opinion between Duesberg, Gallo and Montagnier have never been properly reflected or reported. The consequences have been serious indeed. It is now apparent that people can live with HIV and never progress to AIDS, but for over a decade young men and women, on finding themselves antibody positive, have believed that they will die within ten years. The impact of this diagnosis, backed by the full weight of the medical orthodoxy, has led to countless psychological deaths.

Retrovirology:
A Catalogue of Errors and Mistaken Assumptions

Some time after the War on Cancer, after discoveries became 'inventions' and researchers became entrepreneurs and Big Biology got too expensive to run without Big Business, biomedicine passed the point of being marshalled.

(Barry Werth, June 1988)[11]

When Nixon declared war on cancer in 1971 and the National Cancer Act was passed, the NIH's National Cancer Institute was dominated by virologists. Robert Gallo and colleagues like Howard Temin, David Baltimore and Myron (Max) Essex were there at the ready with millions of dollars at their disposal, ready to find a viral cause for cancer. The intensity and enthusiasm encompassing the field of virology has to be seen in the context of the invention and use of the electron microscope. Its development in the 1940s led to a school of molecular biologists and virologists who were able to probe deeper and deeper into cells, eventually magnifying them up to 50,000 times. What they saw was all new territory, and what they did was ascribe diseases to particles they subsequently identified as retroviruses – *because they were there*. But association has never been proof of causation and research in this field turned into scientific reductionism (*ad absurdum*), which in turn led to a series of monumental mistaken assumptions. Institutional arrogance, unaccountability and staggering displays of greed and vainglory cemented one mistaken hypothesis on to another to form an unassailable construct – the virus/AIDS hypothesis.

Interest in possible cancer causing tumour viruses had been stirred as far back as 1910 when Peyton Rous found he could induce tumours in healthy chickens by inoculating them with tumour tissue from chickens with sarcomas. But no one was able to duplicate Rous's results when they tried to repeat the experiments in other animals. It is Duesberg's view that retroviruses like the Rous sarcoma virus are of little clinical relevance to disease in animals or humans. 'That [virus] has killed probably one chicken outside the laboratory,' he says. 'But there are two Nobel prizes and twelve National Academy of Sciences members for that chicken alone. They don't ever say it that way, but it's true.'[12]

In his book *Virus Hunting*, Gallo gives his own interpretation of what he saw as the noble search for a viral cause for disease. He takes us through the early days of animal retrovirus hunting. Key researchers in the field were Harvard scientist Max Essex, and William Haseltine, who, together with Gallo, led the search for cancer causing retroviruses during the heyday of the cancer campaign. Gallo then moves on to the discovery of oncogenes (incidentally it was Duesberg who identified the first one in his own laboratory).

It was thought that oncogenes might hold the key to all cancers. The oncogene is a special gene, which, when incorporated into the genetic material of a virus, was thought to be able to convert a normal cellular gene into a cancer gene (or cellular oncogene). However, Duesberg, having tested the relationship between cellular and viral genes, pointed out that viral oncogenes are so rare and so artificial that they are not relevant to cancer in humans or wild animals,[13] thereby overturning the main premise of cancer research of the 1970s and 1980s and, as a result, disinviting himself from any of the major scientific conferences on the subject. To date, there have been no major breakthroughs from the oncogene work and no virus has been found that can cause a conventional cancer tumour in humans. Most importantly, there is still no evidence that cancer is an infectious, transmissible disease.

At about the same time (1970) came the discovery of reverse transcriptase activity, which led to the identification of retroviruses. This enzyme enabled an RNA-based virus to knit itself into its host cell's DNA nucleus. No one had believed that this could happen. It was always thought that DNA converted to RNA but not vice versa. This led to the Nobel prize being awarded to Howard Temin and David Baltimore in 1975. Many say Professor Harry Rubin at Berkeley did the important pioneering work on this and should have been recognized for it. All of this spurred Gallo on, he says, 'to look for the first cancer-causing human retrovirus'.[14] But here began a catalogue of calamitous errors that would make even the most dedicated follower of fashion in science shudder. It also lends us a clue as to how other huge 'mistakes', like the mix-up between Montagnier's and Gallo's 'AIDS virus' and the biggest mistake of all – attaching a viral cause for AIDS – came to be made.

The first mistake came hard on the heels of Temin and Baltimore's discovery of reverse transcriptase. When reverse transcriptase was found it was thought to identify retroviral activity and hence infection because retroviruses were known to require reverse transcriptase in order to knit themselves into their host cell. Gallo swiftly announced finding evidence of retroviral infection in human leukaemias. It was described as a 'milestone discovery' because it was the first time evidence had been produced linking retroviruses with disease in humans. Scientists around the world desperately tried to reproduce his discovery but failed. Gallo's critics thought that by linking himself to the work of Temin and Baltimore, he (Gallo) might be heading for a Nobel prize a few years hence,[15] but his 'milestone discovery' was found to be an uncontrolled artefact, in other words a false positive.

The signs of serious overenthusiasm appeared in 1975 when Gallo announced that he had isolated the first human retrovirus from a leukaemia patient. He was all set to discuss his findings at the annual virus cancer programme meeting in Hershey, Pennsylvania and in preparation had sent some samples for independent examination. To his dismay, he heard at the meeting that his human retrovirus was no more than a laboratory contamination of not one, but three different animal retroviruses, from a monkey, a gibbon and a baboon!

Gallo was deeply hurt, and angry enough to suggest that there had been some 'monkey business'. 'I mean, what could it be but sabotage? One contamination can occur, but three? In fifteen years I had had one contamination from a mouse. But three?'[16] This incident prefigures the vehemence with which Gallo initially denied the accusation that his HIV virus was a contaminant from Montagnier's laboratory. Commenting on the Hershey incident, Gallo said:

What surprised me is not the findings – as I say, I was already developing my own doubts – but the vehemence with which they were delivered. More than one speaker used our misfortune to ridicule the very idea of a human retrovirus. It seemed as if a special effort were being made not simply to point out our error but to put the final nails in the coffin of the study of human retroviruses.[17]

After a decade of research and many thousands of millions of dollars, the cancer programme had run aground. The joke running around the laboratories was, 'Human tumour virus? Or human rumour virus?' In 1977, the National Cancer Institute's virus cancer programme was abruptly closed down. Duesberg's epitaph for the programme runs as follows:

When you're in the retrovirus business you can detect a retrovirus. When you look at disease, you can look for the retrovirus. We have done that before with multiple sclerosis, we have done it with sarcomas, and in almost all cases a virus was found sooner or later. What was not emphasized by many of these laboratories was that the same viruses were subsequently always found in healthy carriers and that's why the virus cancer programme is essentially a failure.[18]

What Would Gallo, the King of Virology, and his Courtiers Do Next?

They had tried to find a viral cause for cancers, then breast cancer, then multiple sclerosis and even Alzheimer's disease. All attempts had failed. There they were sitting in their glass and concrete towers twiddling their thumbs. The money had run out, and the Bob Club had begun to disperse. But not for long.

Gallo desperately needed a breakthrough and he finally had one. He took cells from patients with leukaemia, grew them in cell cultures and found reverse transcriptase activity. There had to be a retrovirus there, he reckoned. He called it human T-cell leukaemia virus (HTLV). This became the first of a series of HTLVs (from HTLV-I to HTLV-V) that Gallo gathered together into a family of retroviruses, but not all of them were obedient children. One of them, HTLV-III, which he declared was the cause of AIDS, was particularly wayward. But before we discuss Gallo's 'AIDS virus' we need to understand exactly how HTLV-I gained credence.

In Japan, in 1975, clusters of cases of leukaemia in elderly patients had been noted in the two southern islands. Kiyoshi Takatsuki of Kyoto University called it adult T-cell leukaemia (ATL) and wondered if there might be an infectious cause. Two other scientists, Yorio Hinuma and Isao Miyoshi were also on the trail, and had isolated a retrovirus which Gallo says was identical to his HTLV.

Gallo claims he and his colleagues isolated the first examples of HTLV in 1978/9, and the results were published in 1980. There was a rush of excitement as the same retrovirus was identified in black patients born in the USA and in people from Caribbean countries, South America, Africa and Japan. The leukaemia condition itself, Gallo said, could take from a few years to 40 years to develop, and he began to speculate wildly about the origins of his discovery – that the retrovirus had come from Africa, where it had infected Old World primates and humans and had reached the Americas through the slave trade. He even suggested that Portuguese traders could have taken the retrovirus to Japan in the sixteenth century – via imported slaves and monkeys![19] Gallo clung fiercely to his hypothesis that HTLV-I was capable of causing disease and it is interesting to read the bullying tones he and his colleagues used whenever anyone dared to question his claims.

One fellow scientist, Dr Carlo Croce in Philadelphia had been so bold as to say he thought HTLV-I was an *indirect* cause of leukaemia (his emphasis). A stern rap on the knuckles was fired off to Croce by Gallo in a letter dated 10 February 1986.

Surely if you are aware enough to comment on HTLV-I disease you ought to do it with greater care. Obviously, you speak semantically when you say HTLV-I is an indirect cause of T-cell leukaemia. . . . What is most surprising to me is that your arguments sound straight out of a 'Duesberg performance'. . . . In short, Carlo, I was surprised by the rapidity and zest of making these conclusions. They appear self-serving and are not helpful to you or to the field.[20]

Gallo sent copies of the letter to William Haseltine and others. Haseltine's reply to Gallo is a fine example of how the 'keepers of the received wisdom' stick together, exercising peer pressure to maintain the consensus. 'Dear Bob,' wrote Haseltine, 'I was pleased that you wrote a note to Carlo. ... I hope that Carlo takes your advice to modify his talks appropriately.'[21]

Always remembering that it was from the HTLV (human T-cell leukaemia virus) family that Gallo claimed the AIDS virus had sprung, it is interesting, with the benefit of hindsight, now to reassess the significance of this 'first human retrovirus', HTLV-I, that had risen to fame so quickly. The problem was, and even Gallo admits it, that the same retrovirus could be found in perfectly healthy people. In fact, he himself states that only 1 per cent of people 'infected' with HTLV-I ever developed leukaemia and the latency period could be as long as 40 years.[22] A Japanese study put the incidence of adult T-cell leukaemia in people with antibodies to the virus as low as 0.06 per cent.[23]

As Gallo continued to gather his HTLV family around him – HTLV-II came next and then the infamous HTLV-III (later to be called HIV, much to Gallo's chagrin as it could no longer be included within his HTLV family) – Duesberg's doubts grew in a very big way. As he began to voice his disbelief about the role of retroviruses in disease, some of his colleagues began to listen and he was invited to write his pivotal paper for *Cancer Research*. This article, 'Retroviruses as carcinogens and pathogens: expectations and reality' with its 280 references was published in March 1987[24] and was the first of a series of devastating attacks on the whole field of oncogenes and virus/cancer research, and also of the virus/AIDS hypothesis. Before we tackle Gallo's claims that his discovery, HTLV-III (i.e. HIV) was the cause of AIDS, we must record Duesberg's criticisms of Gallo's earlier assertions that a retrovirus like HTLV-I could cause cancer.

In his *Cancer Research* paper Duesberg describes retroviruses as the most common and benign passenger viruses of healthy animals and humans, probably because of the unique way they have of coexisting with their host cell without causing disease symptoms and also because of the way they can replicate without killing their host cell. He points to the very few cases of leukaemia in animals and humans infected with retroviruses – the risk being as low as 0.1 per cent, which is as low as the risk of leukaemia in animals and people without the virus.

Duesberg goes on to explain that the only role the suspected retroviruses called oncogenes play in cancer is to cause abnormal cells to be made (hyperplasia) which are not necessarily malignant. The only way this abnormal accumulation of cells can occur is when the virus is forced into highly concentrated levels in 'hothouse' laboratory conditions. Hardly ever has an animal outside the laboratory developed a malignant cancer from these viruses and never has there been a reported case of a human developing cancer from them. He concludes by saying that latent retroviruses are almost always involved in all natural infections but they do not, either directly or indirectly, cause cancer tumours. They are simply passengers and should not be regarded as targets for cancer prevention or cancer therapy.[25]

After publication of his article, Duesberg was interviewed by author John Lauritsen. Duesberg told him he did not think HTLV-I played any role at all in leukaemias. He emphasized his point that only in laboratories, where animals are forced by injecting high quantities of virus into them before they have properly developed their own immune system to resist this assault, do they produce abnormal cells.[26]

Although most of the *Cancer Research* article challenged the accepted view on the relationship of retroviruses to cancer, the last section led on to challenge the virus/AIDS hypothesis. Duesberg's key points were that the level of HIV in the body, even in advanced AIDS was too low to cause disease; that a retrovirus like HIV was not capable of killing its host cell and going on to infect others; that the latency period did not make sense, because viruses cause infection when they enter the body and cannot wait five or ten years before they cause harm; and that the cases of AIDS without HIV and HIV without AIDS made a nonsense of infectious virus/AIDS hypothesis.

These important points had never been put before, yet here they were, published in a prestigious scientific journal. After studying them carefully we became convinced that we should pursue these lines of argument further. It was this article, first spotted by my colleague Jad Adams, that changed the course of our lives, and set our small team off on a ten-year quest to document one of the most fascinating battles ever, at the leading edge of science.

Gallo Links HTLV-III to AIDS

The idea that AIDS might be caused by a retrovirus was circulating as far back as 1981. All the early cases of AIDS were identified by the fact that young men with symptoms of AIDS shared a common factor, their T-cell count was very low. T-cells are a subset of white blood cells that are crucial to the immune system. By 1982, after hearing James Curran of the Centers for Disease Control describe cases of young men with a very low T-cell count and express the view that they might be looking at the first signs of a newly emerging and potentially epidemic disease, bells began to ring in Gallo's head. What could be affecting these T-cells, he wondered? 'Intellectually, I began to play out one scenario. What if AIDS were due to a mutation of an HTLV, probably occurring in Africa, which had spread to Haiti, then to the United States?'[27]

Gallo's friend Max Essex had already been working on the idea that if HTLV-I could infect T-cells and cause leukaemia, why couldn't it also cause another disease during its (alleged) long period of latency? As AIDS reportedly affected T-cells, why couldn't HTLV-I also cause AIDS? It was from then on that AIDS, which until then had been just a collection of disparate symptoms, began to be labelled as a single disease with a single infectious cause. Once the word 'infectious' was introduced all the epidemic-control alarm bells were set off at once. The problem was that if HTLV-I were supposed to cause infected cells to multiply and grow into cancers, how could it at the same time kill T-cells off? 'Indeed,' write Peter Duesberg and Bryan Ellison:

Retroviruses had seized the high ground of cancer research in the 1970s precisely because they did not kill infected cells, but rather integrated themselves into the cell's cancer-causing agents. Still, Essex's hypothesis, implicating HTLV-I appealed to Gallo – until he finally noticed the contra-diction. Gallo then quietly changed the name of the virus; for Human T-cell Leukaemia Virus he substituted Human T-cell Lymphotropic Virus, meaning one that favours infecting T-cells [or T-Lymphocytes]. This new name implied neither cancer nor cell-killing, thereby maintaining an ambiguity that could allow the virus to cause both diseases at once.[28]

In other words Gallo, realizing that HTLV-I had been associated with the cell proliferation necessary to cause a cancer like leukaemia, now had to explain how the retrovirus he claimed to have discovered could work in an opposite way and kill cells off. He simply distanced HTLV-I from leukaemia by substituting the 'L' for leukaemia in HTLV-I to 'L' for lymphotropic. Lymphotropic means a preference for T-lymphocytes, which allowed Gallo to cover all his options. Gallo and his co-workers set about testing the blood of patients with AIDS and, after enormous efforts to find a cell line they could work with as well as pooling ten different retroviruses into one brew (a technique that has been highly criticized by fellow scientists), Gallo came up with a new retrovirus he duly kept in the family and named HTLV-III. It was now 1984.

In the meantime, at the Pasteur Institute in Paris, Montagnier and his co-workers had also been busy isolating a virus strain from a young man with swollen lymph nodes. They came up with a retrovirus they cautiously named LAV (lymphadenopathy associated virus). Gallo encouraged them to write up their results and in April 1983 he sent Montagnier's paper to the journal *Science*. Montagnier had been in touch with Gallo, and Gallo had offered to look through the paper before its publication. Montagnier had not written an abstract for the paper, so Gallo offered to write it for him and read it to him over the telephone. Gallo had written the following lines, 'We report here the isolation of a novel retrovirus from the lymph node of a homosexual patient with multiple lymphadenopathies. The virus appears to be a member of the human T-cell leukaemia virus (HTLV) family.'[29] This last sentence was to reverberate through history. Montagnier claimed later that he had not fully understood Gallo's English on the telephone and would never have accepted Gallo's linking LAV to his HTLV family.[30] None the less, in July 1983, Montagnier brought Gallo samples of LAV together with a set of his photographs.

Oddly enough, no one had taken much notice of Montagnier's 1983 paper in *Science*. Then, in the spring of 1984, word got out that Gallo had finally tracked down the cause of AIDS. It was Gallo's own HTLV-III. As a result, a most unusual thing happened. Before the publication of any information about HTLV-III and AIDS to the scientific community, a press conference was called. Margaret Heckler, Secretary of the Department of Health and Human Services, with Gallo by her side declared, 'The probable cause of AIDS has been found.' On the same day Gallo filed a US patent for the HIV blood test kit he had developed.

Dr Kary Mullis, who was awarded the 1993 Nobel prize for chemistry for inventing polymerase chain reaction, a method of DNA/RNA amplification, subsequently used to detect HIV in blood samples, shakes his head when he remembers that day.

Why they did it I cannot figure out. Nobody in their right mind would jump into this thing like they did. The secretary of health just announcing to the world like that that this man Robert Gallo, wearing those dark sunglasses, had found the cause of AIDS. It had nothing to do with any well-considered science. There were some people who had AIDS and some of them had HIV not even all of them. So they had a correlation. So what?[31]

Mullis is equally scathing about Montagnier's labelling of his isolate, from the lymph node of a homosexual man, as the cause of AIDS.

Just because someone who needed to find a clinical connection with a virus belonging to the only type of virus he knew how to work with, found one of them in a patient who had a new disease that was beginning to play a role in medicine, he blamed it [the virus] as the cause... Do you see how it works? ... Anyone looking into this would say this man had a personal interest in finding a link between his own virus and this disease. Did Montagnier investigate all known viruses, and then finally, for some good reason, home in on this one? Because, if he had looked for any other virus in that lymph node, he would have found it. And that was already in the literature.[32]

From the day of the Washington press conference, the virus/AIDS hypothesis became gospel and the money started to flow. Gallo received $100,000 a year from the test patent. William Haseltine, one of Gallo's close working colleagues in the darker days of retrovirus-linked cancer research, had formed a biotechnology company called Cambridge Bioscience and invited Max Essex to join him. This suited Essex well, from his position at Harvard's School of Public Health. Although Harvard would own the patents on any-thing he discovered, Cambridge Bioscience would have the licence, which is where the real money was made. 'Thus it [Harvard] would have a vested interest in what research Essex chose to give priority to and how he assigned graduate students to experiments. It was a blur-ring of business and education,' wrote Barry Werth in *New England Monthly*. Essex had connected HTLV with AIDS a year before the putative cause of AIDS was identified and he clung to his theory even after the discovery of HIV.

His reluctance to consider the doubts about his work raised concern over his role in AIDS from the start – and not only his role. Other researchers began suspecting Essex, Gallo and Haseltine of having their own agenda to promote the particular family of retroviruses first found by Gallo. This was said to explain Gallo's attempts to have the AIDS virus named HTLV-III.[33]

Needless to say, when HIV and AIDS became big business, Essex and Haseltine became millionaires, despite yet another monumental blunder on Essex's part. He was investigating two AIDS-related viruses, one in African monkeys and one in apparently healthy prostitute women in Senegal. These 'new' virus isolates were, of course, quickly patented. But then a young Harvard scientist called Barry Mullins discovered that both of the much talked about 'new' AIDS-related viruses were no more than contaminants from domestic monkey viruses that were being worked on in an upstairs laboratory! 'Congratu-lations!' exclaimed my colleague Michael Verney-Elliott, 'The people who did not bring you the cause of cancer have now not brought you the cause of AIDS.'

The Fight to Claim HIV's Discovery

Meanwhile, in Paris, Luc Montagnier was not a happy man. Not only had Gallo claimed his virus isolate, now HTLV-III (later renamed HIV), was the cause of AIDS but he had published a photograph of Montag-nier's virus in a *Science* article announcing his (Gallo's) findings. Then, to add insult to injury, Gallo had applied for a US patent for the

AIDS blood test based on HTLV-III when Montagnier had applied for an LAV-based patent a year and a half earlier, and it had not yet been granted.

Montagnier was incensed, and at the end of 1985 he, together with the Pasteur Institute, decided to sue the US government. 'I was particularly furious that our patent for the blood test was ignored until Gallo's was accepted. Scientists in the US are exposed to high pressure to produce results, and it sometimes warps their sense of ethics. Scientists have even faked their experiments to look like winners and not only in the US.'[34] The story of how the AIDS virus mix-up occurred has been amply documented, in particular by John Crewdson of the *Chicago Tribune*, whose painstaking research and subsequent article, that filled a whole supplement of the *Chicago Tribune*, led to an official investigation of Gallo's work (see Chapter 11).[35]

Gallo's HTLV-III turned out to be identical to Montagnier's LAV (later it was agreed that both be renamed HIV) and the only conclusion that could be drawn was that somehow Montagnier's virus had contaminated Gallo's laboratory cultures, and Gallo admitted as much in his 1991 letter to *Nature*.[36] At a time when the public was calling for urgent funding for AIDS research, it would have been embarrassing for the French and US governments to be seen to be locked into a hugely expensive legal battle about test kit patent revenue, so at the behest of President Ronald Reagan and French Prime Minister Jacques Chirac, Gallo and Montagnier met in a Frankfurt hotel room to work out a settlement. The end result was that the French and Americans settled the lawsuit. In March 1987, they agreed to share the credit for discovering the virus and split the royalties from the blood test kits. By 1994 those royalties had amounted to $35 million.[37]

Gallo and Montagnier would be bound by an agreed 'scientific history' of events. This 'history' was published in *Nature*. No mention is made of laboratory contamination or dates when respective patents were applied for, simply that in May 1983 Montagnier's group reported the identification of a 'novel human retrovirus' LAV, cultured from a patient with the AIDS syndrome. And that in May 1984 Gallo's group reported finding HTLV-III in AIDS patients (and claimed it was the cause of AIDS). It was agreed that both retroviruses LAV and HTLV-III should be given the same name – human immunodeficiency virus – HIV.[38] The text of the agreement between Gallo and Montagnier contains a clause whereby the two parties agree not to, 'make nor publish any statement which would or could be construed as contradicting or compromising the integrity of the said scientific history.'[39] Jad Adams, an historian himself, is dismayed at this 'fixed' interpretation of events. 'If scientific fraud is the worst professional crime a scientist can conceive of, probably the worst for a historian is the rewriting of history to accommodate some establishment view.'[40]

Gallo has shrugged off the controversy surrounding Luc Montagnier's claim that Gallo used his isolate to make a commercial AIDS test. He says it has had no impact on his reputation, 'Every one in the scientific community knows my study, and they know we were not found guilty of anything.'[41] Today, having left the NIH after being vilified by the *Chicago Tribune*, and targeted by three separate investigations (see below and Chapter 11), Gallo has managed to re-establish himself as head of his new Institute of Human Virology, at the University of Maryland, Baltimore, where he continues with his research.

Gallo holds 13 US patents and has applied for 29 others. His inventions have brought his previous employers, the NIH, half of its income from royalties. The University of Maryland will hold the patents on new inventions emerging from Gallo's Institute of Human Virology, but will split the profits fifty-fifty with the inventors. Great hopes are pinned on Gallo. If he is successful, his institute is expected to become self-supporting within five years and the state of Maryland stands to make millions in spin-offs. However, there have been some doubts. When the Maryland legislature agreed to fund Gallo's institute it pointedly added an ethics clause requiring the university to vouch for the institute's behaviour. 'Privately, some faculty members at the university admit to having similar reservations about their new neighbour,' writes Elaine Richman in *The Sciences*. 'They fear that spectres from Gallo's past will return to haunt them, or that his new institute will drain away state funds for salaries and research.'[42]

Expectations are high that Gallo will discover a cure for AIDS. He is currently working on three naturally occurring substances that appear to be able to halt replication of HIV by locking it out of cells. These substances are described as HIV-suppressive factors (HIV-SF) and belong to a class of compounds called chemokines.

Gallo's most recent foray into the public arena was at the 1997 meeting of the American Association for the Advancement of Science where he announced his work into the treatment of Kaposi's sarcoma lesions with a protein linked to a hormone found in the urine of pregnant women. In one unpublished European trial, Gallo said the hormone product apparently killed the AIDS virus in terminally ill patients. In typical Gallo-speak, he warns, 'We still know too little about this stuff. . . . We haven't sequenced its chemical structure. We don't know the doses to use, or the route for administering it. But we do have a hope that we've found a new nontoxic weapon against AIDS.'[43]

Goings on in Gallo's Laboratory: Laboratory Colleagues are Convicted

When a scientist achieves fame and renown such as that accorded to Robert Gallo, the general press prefers to sustain the glowing accolades rather than report on any unsavoury events surrounding the hero. Between 1988 and 1991 Gallo's laboratory at the NIH was in a state of upheaval. Gallo himself had come under investigation by the US government's Office of Research Integrity, by the office of Democratic representative John Dingell and by a special panel appointed by the National Academy of Sciences. Three of his closest associates at his laboratory came under criminal investigation involving fraud and embezzlement. Although the US press covered some of these events, the following stories were not picked up by the international press. Who wants to knock a hero off his pedestal? But the succession of investigations must leave a question mark as to the ethics of a man who can work so closely with people who were eventually found guilty and convicted of dishonest business practices involving his own (Gallo's) laboratory.

In the late 1980s, morale at the Gallo laboratory was at a low ebb. One of Gallo's top associates, NIH staff researcher Syed Zaki Salahuddin, came under criminal investigation in 1989 for being involved with a company called Pan-Data Systems that was selling virus samples allegedly removed from Gallo's laboratory at the NIH. Among the charges raised concerning Salahuddin was that he 'purchased supplies at the NIH store using the credit card assigned to Gallo's laboratory; these were then delivered to Pan-Data Systems' new laboratory'. Moreover, 'A Pan-Data Systems employee made products in Salahuddin's section of Gallo's laboratory that Pan-Data Systems then sold to other biomedical firms.'[44] Another of Gallo's laboratory associates, Dr Dharam Ablashi was also implicated in promoting these sales. The virus samples involved were HTLV-I, HTLV-II and the so-called AIDS virus HTLV-III, which sold for about $1000 a milligram. Pan-Data was also selling the HIV test kit at a reduced price.

Salahuddin was found guilty and sentenced to repay $12,000 and to carry out 1750 hours of community service. Yet, he was a major author in the papers announcing the discovery of the AIDS virus, as was Gallo's second-in-command at the laboratory, Prem Sarin. Sarin also found himself on trial for embezzlement – for paying $25,000 into his private account that should have gone towards hiring a laboratory technician. He was fired by the NIH. All in all there were four inquiries into Gallo's laboratory in 1990. Duesberg would throw his hands up saying he could not understand why no one dared question Gallo's position on AIDS even when it became known he had had two convicted felons working closely with him for years.[45]

By 1990 Gallo was in trouble again. A major NIH investigation was set up to look into his collaboration with French scientist Daniel Zagury. The project was to test 19 African volunteers with a supposed AIDS vaccine. Three of the volunteers died, but neither Zagury nor Gallo reported these deaths to the French or US regulatory authorities that govern such experiments. A published account of the research by the French and American scientists collaborating on the project made no mention of the deaths in spite of the fact that at the time the article appeared, two subjects had died. French government records show that nearly three months after the first death, the study was expanded to include more subjects.[46] In their defence, the French team claimed there was no cover-up but that they did not announce the deaths because the patients did not belong to the group being studied and were accepted into the trial on compassionate grounds.

By a strange coincidence, Gallo reported a burglary at his home soon after the Zagury paper was published and word of the cover-up got out. The burglar left the family jewellery and silverware intact. According to Gallo, only one thing had been disturbed – some scientific data sent to him by Zagury. Gallo named *Chicago Tribune* journalist John Crewdson as his main suspect. (Crewdson had written the major exposé on the Montagnier/Gallo dispute about the discovery of HIV.) The police investigation was eventually dropped.[47] These events may seem trivial and unconnected with the grand theme of HIV and AIDS, but they are important to document because the general public has no notion of how Big Science can so easily become corrupted and, when huge sums of money are at stake, Big Ideas with little or no scientific basis can so easily become the accepted orthodoxy. In an extraordinarily coy display Gallo sums up his attitude to the possibility that his virus may have been a contaminant from Montagnier's laboratory. In a small footnote towards the end of his book he writes:

Later I had reasons to think that if the two viruses were so closely related that they might have been mixed up (accidental contamination), the mix-up would likely have occurred in my laboratory. In any case, because we had many other isolates and had made several other key scientific advances, not to mention the enormous scientific-medical problems that still lay ahead of us, my co-workers and I did not think this likelihood terribly important.[48]

There was of course only the small matter of the patent for the blood test at stake with its attendant millions of dollars! The question that may never be solved is whether or not the 'mix-up' was an accident or (to put it charitably) a succession of events dictated by blind ambition and arrogance.

It was in May 1991 that *Nature* published the letter from Gallo admitting that the virus he had announced in 1984 was not a new discovery, and that his researchers had, whether mistakenly or deliberately, used it as the basis for the American breakthrough.[49] When Montagnier was asked to comment he told reporters in Paris, 'I feel a certain relief at the end of this seven-year quarrel. But I think that at a certain moment there was a lie.' There is a strange irony in Gallo's choice of a quote for his book, from Sandra Panem's *The AIDS Bureaucracy*. In an attempt to exculpate himself, he tries to make the end justify the means. What he sees as a virtue – his decision in 1984 (regardless of the row about whose virus was whose) to focus entirely on HIV as the cause of AIDS – is precisely the vice that overwhelmed the entire scientific establishment. Gallo quotes Panem as follows:

Regardless of the political [Gallo's emphasis] *settlement concerning who discovered the AIDS virus* [Gallo notes: and, of course, the development of the blood test, by inference], *and who will garner Nobel prizes or public opprobrium, the May 1984 acceptance of HTLV-III/LAV as the cause of AIDS irreversibly changed the nature of managing the epidemic. Prior to that time AIDS research was groping: now it had direction. Scientists could go on to real targeting of specific tests and treatments and prevention strategies. Whereas coordination and augmented resources had always been desirable, they now became mandatory. And so the debate over research management strategies as well as questions of public policy was dramatically changed.*[50]

Those were dramatic changes indeed. They set the world off on a course of plague terror and they lulled drug users and the fast lane members of the gay community into a false sense of security, blaming an external source for their ills and relying on condoms and clean needles for their salvation – which sadly never came.

Chapter 5

Plague Terror

Fuelling the Plague Terror Machine

I t is June 1995 and articles, faxes and E-mail continue to stream through our office about the AIDS debate. Two articles published in the same week of June catch my eye. The first is an Internet communication with the text of a front-page article in the *Sunday Telegraph* by Victoria Macdonald, with the headline 'AIDS tide has turned in Europe, claims professor'. The article reads:

The multi-billion pound AIDS industry is in turmoil over claims by the French scientist who discovered the HIV virus in 1983 that the disease has stabilized and is even declining in parts of northern Europe. Professor Luc Montagnier, president of the World Foundation for AIDS Research and Prevention, has delivered a blow to patient organizations, saying the problem is currently most severe in Africa and Asia and that efforts should now be concentrated there. In an interview with the Sunday Telegraph, *Prof. Montagnier said it was time the public was told the truth. He said there was no 'explosion' of AIDS in northern Europe, adding it was wrong to frighten the general public into thinking that there was a high risk of catching the disease because it only caused a backlash when it did not appear.*[1]

The second fax, also dated June 1995, was an article from the *New York Times*. The headline read, 'White House apologizes for rubber gloves' and continued:

White House police officers were wrong to put on rubber gloves before admitting a delegation of gay elected officials, President Clinton's spokes-

man said today. ... About 40 visitors, who included state senators and representatives and other elected officials, were met by members of the uniformed division of the Secret Service, many of them wearing rubber gloves. The officials raised the incident at the meeting saying, 'medical authorities say the virus is not transmitted by casual contact' and several of the visitors said they were offended by the action.[2]

Two details within these articles should be noted. Montagnier's interest in focusing on AIDS in the Third World was no accident. He was building a laboratory in the Ivory Coast's capital, Abidjan, where he proposed to do research work with HIV-positive blood samples from the local population. Although Montagnier had shifted away from the HIV = AIDS = death formula, had admitted that 'some strains of HIV' may not cause AIDS and had denounced panic about a heterosexual spread of AIDS in Europe, he was still committed to HIV as the main cause of AIDS. Perhaps he could do little else whatever his doubts, for the Pasteur Institute where he worked had now become dependent on the revenue from its patented HIV test kits.

The other point helps to understand the total conviction with which people speak of HIV as the undisputed cause of AIDS. Notice the *New York Times*'s phrase, 'the officers apparently were concerned about being infected by the HIV, the virus that causes AIDS.' It had become axiomatic that every reference to HIV was followed up by this apparently valid explanation.

These two articles in the very same week of 1995 demonstrated the confused atmosphere of conflicting propaganda that had built up over the preceding decade. Sloppy scientific articles hypothesizing about what HIV could and could not do, dramatic claims about 'breakthroughs' in controlling the virus which have come to nothing, combined with vast financial interests and the desire to be 'politically correct' when confronted by those gay lobbyists who persisted in clinging to HIV as the source of all their ills, had produced a powerful cocktail of misinformation, the most lethal ingredient of which was the plague–terror machine.

Fear of plague is as old as mankind, and there are those who know how to exploit it only too well – politicians, pharmaceutical companies, journalists, public health officials and organizations like the US Epidemic Intelligence Service (EIS) (about which more later). A random collection of media reports over a decade gives ample proof of how the plague terror machine has been put to work on AIDS – some laughable, some poignant and some unbearably tragic. In the *Independent* of 25 July 1989, we have a snippet of foreign news entitled 'AIDS and polygamy'.

Zimbabwean polygamists are being warned by the government not to use the fear of AIDS as an excuse to divorce their unwanted wives. The message was conveyed by Samuel Makanza, the provincial medical superintendent for Manicaland, where many peasants practise polygamy. However, he did urge them to restrain themselves and not to acquire any new ones. . . . There are only 321 confirmed cases of AIDS in Zimbabwe.

Jumping back to the *Sunday Times*, of November 1986, we find an article by Peter Wilshire and Neville Hodgkinson. (Hodgkinson has bravely challenged the virus/AIDS hypothesis in recent years but readily admits that he, too, was caught up in the frenzy of early AIDS panic.) The article has a huge headline 'AT RISK' and quotes a report from the US National Academy of Sciences warning that if the virus is not checked 'the present epidemic could become a catastrophe'. The article continues in further tones of doom, 'There is no reason to expect significant differences between the British and the US experience. . . . The UK is moving steadily up exactly the same escalator as the Americans. Unless the disease can be halted, or at least contained, we too face the prospect that 10,000 people will die from AIDS-related diseases before the end of the decade.'[3]

Actually, at the end of July 1989, the cumulative figure for AIDS deaths in the UK was 1523, from a cumulative total of registered AIDS cases of 2343. The deaths constituted 65 per cent of the total. By the end of 1990, from 4068 registered AIDS cases, the figure for deaths was 2645 (still 65 per cent).

Wilshire and Hodgkinson include a side column in their spread where they list some 'old wives tales about how the affliction can be spread'. 'Many can be immediately nailed', they write:

AIDS *cannot be caught from barber's scissors, coughing in public, garbage collected at a lesbian social centre, or shaking hands with a known carrier (all of which have figured in various recent outbursts of hysteria). But others, like the wholly unsubstantiated suggestion that* AIDS *started with a disastrous bungle in genetic engineering, are almost impossible to disprove.*

The trickiest involve saliva, from which it has been possible to culture virus, though in far smaller quantities than in blood or semen, the normal vehicles of transmission. Even tears and breast-milk have not been cleared entirely. So there is at least a remote chance of infection through such activities as kissing, mouth-to-mouth resuscitation, dentistry, drinking from the communion chalice, or even, it has been suggested, trying out an unsterilized contact lens.[4]

The *Guardian*, 22 October 1986: 'Kiss of life woman may have AIDS'. 'Scotland Yard wants to trace a young woman who may have contracted AIDS after giving the kiss of life to a road accident victim in north London last week. Police believe the injured man who died later, may have been an AIDS carrier.' The *Guardian*, 15 March 1990: 'Bathers "face AIDS risk" from sewage'. 'Swimmers on beaches contaminated by raw sewage outfalls could risk catching the AIDS virus, HIV, MPs were told yesterday. New tests have shown that the virus could live for more than 24 hours if pumped into the sea through sewage outfalls. Although the risk is remote, a swimmer with an open sore could be infected.'

But as usual it is John Lauritsen who takes the prize for capturing the mood in his 4 July 1988 piece for the *New York Native* called 'Latex Lunacy'. 'Events have gone beyond satire,' he writes:

On June 1st, an American company, Hemodynamics Inc., announced that it would soon receive the first shipment of a total of 18 million latex gloves from a Malaysian corporation with which it has formed a joint venture. Hemodynamics attributed the demand for the latex gloves to concern over the so-called 'AIDS virus' and its impact on the health care profession. Hemodynamics expects that the Malaysian latex venture will add $10 million to its revenues.

Latex gloves have acquired talismanic properties; they symbolize protection against the evil virus akin to such medieval charms as garlic flowers,

crucifixes, amulets or magic gestures. . . . Another form of latex, the con-
dom, is being promoted as the panacea for AIDS *prevention, as the premier*
symbol of 'safe sex'. AIDS *groups, 'gay leaders', church groups, public*
health departments, colleges and Surgeon General Koop have all joined in
the chorus of praise for condoms. At Dartmouth, an official student group,
RAID (Responsible AIDS *Information at Dartmouth), put on an exhibition*
of safe sex, in which a male student held a plunger between his legs and a
female student slid a condom over the handle. Then students did timed
contests to see who could place condoms on dildos the fastest.

Lauritsen asks:

Is AIDS *truly an epidemic? In terms of numbers* AIDS *does not qualify for*
an epidemic. In a decade, from 1978 to the present, there have been only
35,188 deaths in the United States from AIDS *complications, out of a*
population of 250 million people. In a true epidemic such as the influenza
epidemic of 1918, more people than that died in a day.[5]

  Two publications from San Francisco are worthy of an entry,
although the repercussions from such childish misinformation are no
laughing matter as people, distracted by the safe sex arguments, neglect the true causes that put them at risk. A gay publication, the *Hot 'n*
Healthy Times, published by Eroticus Publications, has a front-page
piece entitled 'Condoms Stop AIDS Virus'. 'Researchers at the University of California, San Francisco, recently proved in laboratory tests
that condoms can stop the AIDS virus. The virus cannot penetrate the
condom material of either latex or natural skin condoms unless the
condoms are ruptured.'[6] Even when condoms are used conventionally
in vaginal intercourse, they have a failure rate of about 10 per cent.
When used for anal intercourse they can break as often as 50 per cent
of the time. On the back page of the same paper there is a column
called 'Safe Sex Guidelines':

'Unsafe – rimming, fisting, blood contact, sharing sex toys or needles,
semen or urine in mouth, anal intercourse without condom, vaginal inter-
course without condom.

57

Possibly safe – *French kissing (wet), anal intercourse with condom, vaginal intercourse with condom, sucking – stop before climax, cunnilingus, watersports external only.*

Safe – *Massage, hugging, mutual masturbation, social kissing (dry), body-to-body rubbing, fantasy voyeurism, exhibitionism.*[7]

It would be funny were it not so sad. This preoccupation with 'safe' and 'unsafe' is ludicrous and yet all the time the young men reading that paper are more than likely taking cocktails of five or six different chemicals every night before 'trying to do it right'.

The fact remains that AIDS has remained firmly within the high risk groups, affecting certain very sexually active gay men and intravenous and recreational drug users, yet most AIDS information for drug users has been almost an incitement to go on taking them. The San Francisco AIDS Foundation published a press release in May 1987, *The Works: Drugs, Sex and AIDS*, 'an informational comic book created for the i.v. [intravenous] drug-using population. ... The colourful, 36-page comic book contains five different stories ... *The Works* vignettes are written at first and third grade levels in vernacular familiar to the needle using community. ... *The Works* addresses the needs of the i.v. drug users.' There is only one mention in the press release about 'the need to avoid needle using' and an accompanying overview says, 'What is the purpose of the comic book? To warn i.v. drug users of the risk of contracting AIDS through sharing needles, and to promote the use of bleach to clean syringes if sharing does take place.'[8]

Nothing about what actually goes through the needles straight into their veins. Nothing about the way these unknown, illegally obtained substances they are injecting three times a day have been adulterated with toxic trash like aflatoxins several times *en route* from Cali or Calcutta. And nothing about the devastating effects these poisons can have on their already overloaded immune systems. The build-up of fear was relentless during the mid to late 1980s. When a report appeared in the *New England Journal of Medicine* in 1989[9] of a prolonged period between HIV infection and detection of antibodies, it posed huge ethical problems for orthopaedic surgeons using bone grafts from deceased road accident victims. How could they know whether the bone they were using was from someone who was in the 'window' or 'limbo' period between infection and seroconversion?

Young couples getting married who thought they should each be tested found later that even if they were HIV negative, they were being refused a mortgage simply because they had *had* an HIV test. In the state of Illinois mandatory premarital HIV tests were introduced in 1988. It was a total failure. The Department of Public Health simply found that couples either went to other states to get married or chose not to marry at all. Further research revealed that during the six month AIDS screening programme, only 8 of 70,846 applicants for a marriage licence were identified as seropositive, and most of those reported a history of risk behaviour. The programme cost $1.5 million.

The World Health Organization (WHO) fed the frenzy. In 1989 Dr Jonathan Mann of the WHO's global programme on AIDS predicted new waves of AIDS cases. He said three times as many cases were expected in the next ten years as had occurred in the 1980s. In November 1989, 187,000 cases of AIDS from 152 countries had been officially reported to the WHO, but the real number of cases world-wide was estimated at 600,000. By the year 2000, six million people may have AIDS, said Mann. It was dangerous to believe comfortable and comforting myths in the face of a worldwide epidemic as fatal as any the world had ever known.[10] By June 1990, at the San Francisco World AIDS conference the WHO was quoting an estimated figure of 15–20 million people infected with HIV by the year 2000.[11]

The figures quoted by the WHO, as we shall see later in a chapter on Africa, were 'bumped up' by hundreds of thousands of presumptive diagnoses in Third World countries where AIDS is diagnosed without an HIV test. In the early 1990s, the WHO's global programme on AIDS was employing between two and three thousand people. They continually fed highly inflated figures to the press, and officials at public meetings began to quote their estimated cases for AIDS in order to drum up funding, quietly dropping the actual reported figures. We challenged these figures at a meeting at the London School of Hygiene and Tropical Medicine in 1993, and there was a red-faced acknowledgement that the figures they were using as fact, were no more than guesswork. In April 1995 the WHO's Global AIDS Programme dismissed some 750 of its workers because none of the 'pandemic' predictions had come true. AIDS had not spread into the heterosexual community in the West and AIDS had not ravaged Third World countries.

Another notable prophet of doom was Professor Roy Anderson of Imperial College in London. His pessimistic view was that a 'second wave' of the disease will appear in drug users in five to ten years, and a 'third wave' among heterosexuals in about 20 to 30 years.[12] In 1988, excited predictions of an advancing spread of heterosexual AIDS used figures for babies born with AIDS in New York as an example to demonstrate that the threat of AIDS was as much of a danger to heterosexuals as to homosexuals in Western society.[13] What was not mentioned was that 80 per cent of the so-called HIV infected babies in the USA were born to drug addicted mothers, including crack addicts who had never injected. These fearful predictions of heterosexual spread were not born out by the facts. In 1989, according to figures published by the Department of Health and Social Security, the total number of cases traced to heterosexual transmission in the UK was 19 (up from 7 in mid-1987). These would normally be described as a 180 per cent increase in heterosexual spread, but the actual figures are insignificant or could be ascribed to misdiagnoses.

Fuel was added to the fire by statements made at the Fifth International AIDS conference quoting 1.5 million Americans with HIV, or 1 in every 250 infected with HIV.[14] But these figures were out of context because the 1.5 million figure (which was an estimate) had remained static since 1983. It had always been the CDC's estimate of HIV positives in the USA and it had not changed. Then, in 1995 they reviewed the figures downwards by 50 per cent and quoted 700,000–800,000 instead. Hardly the sign of a raging, infectious pandemic. There were many other examples of panic statistics. Figures taken in 1989 from the UK government's Office of Population Censuses and Surveys, which in turn were based on the most modest of a set of six assumptions produced by the Institute of Actuaries, predicted that 100,000 men would die of AIDS in the next ten years in England and Wales and that 200,000 would die over the next 30 years.[15] By

September 1996 there had been 9447 deaths from AIDS in England and Wales. To fulfil the 1999 prediction (of 100,000 deaths), 90,553 men would have to die within three years!

There was no real challenge to these statements and no one openly questioned the wisdom of accepting information from organizations issuing figures that were clearly wildly inflated on the basis of the evidence available at that time. Alarm, dismay and bad science continued to fan the flames of plague terror. Doctors and scientists who should have known better were just as much, if not more, to blame as the media. Take the case of presumed mother-to-child transmission of HIV. A huge European collaborative study was set up to monitor mother-to-child transmission of HIV under Professor Catherine Peckham at the Institute of Child Health in London. A report of the study in the *Lancet* in November 1988 described how 271 children born to HIV-infected mothers had been followed up in eight European centres for over a year. Only ten had developed AIDS, and the article stated that 'most children in the European study were born to mothers who abused intravenous drugs.'[16] Long before HIV ever came on the map it was well-known that babies born to drug-using mothers were frequently born prematurely, underweight, with small head circumference, showing failure to thrive and a severely compromised immune system, which often led to the infant's death.

However, such was the panic surrounding HIV positive mothers that there had been calls for termination of pregnancy or sterilization for all seropositive women. Luckily the call was not heeded, but many HIV positive women will have experienced agonies of indecision as to whether or not to have a child. Fear also led many HIV positive women to stop breastfeeding their children, even though there was no evidence that HIV was transmitted in breast milk. This brings to mind the remark made by New York physician and pioneering AIDS dissident, Dr Joseph Sonnabend, to reporter Roger Rapaport in Oakland, California's *Sunday Tribune*:

Finding an organism doesn't mean it is linked to a disease. In the 1970s scientists produced a model of a mouse mammary tumour virus. They then found particles of a similar retrovirus in human breast cancer patients.

Afraid that the women could transmit the virus through breast milk, they advised the women to stop breastfeeding. Then it was discovered that many healthy women had the same retrovirus. As a result no one took the suggestion seriously. It is the same problem with the HIV/AIDS link.[17]

But the scientific community had begun to clutch at straws. In 1988, Michael Haseltine, one of the 'Bob [Gallo] Club', suggested that all healthy individuals at risk could be given a daily, low dose 'chemical vaccine' of AZT.[18] Given the known toxicity of AZT, this can only be described as desperation medicine.

Vague and unfocused suppositions dressed up as 'Science' by AIDS pundits were given free reign in the press. 'Major breakthroughs' were constantly reported. The HIV virus could be 'halted' or 'neutralized', we would hear. A protein molecule had been created in the laboratory that could render the AIDS virus non-infectious.[19] But nothing was heard about these breakthroughs again. For example, in January 1989, Gallo announced 'a major breakthrough' at the Venice International Symposium on Cancer Research and AIDS. He was reported as saying that an exciting development in the understanding of virus replication could mean that within five years it should be possible to control the spread of the virus in HIV-infected people. The breakthrough involved developing drugs that would inhibit the process that allowed the virus to get out of its cell and go on to infect others. Theoretically, if the inhibitor could be perfected, the infected person would not be able to pass the infection on to anyone else.[20]

This can only be described as make-believe science. The number of 'ifs', 'maybes', and phrases like 'could theoretically' abound in Gallo's language. The irresponsibility of making these announcements to the press without any real scientific evidence led to an escalation of plague terror that even Luc Montagnier found necessary to damp down.

AIDS Panic: The HIV Witchhunt

Who would have believed that fear of plague, infection and contamination could lead to a twentieth century version of medieval witch hunts? It happened in Arcadia, Florida in 1987. The Ray family have four children, three boys and a girl. The three boys, Ricky aged 10, Robert 9 and Randy 8, have haemophilia and were found to be HIV positive. It was thought at the time that their antibody positive state resulted from their injections of Factor VIII, the blood clotting factor they needed to avoid haemorrhages. The three boys had no symptoms of AIDS, yet in the autumn of 1986 they were barred from Memorial Elementary School, DeSoto County. When a federal judge ordered their reinstatement, a local group called Citizens Against AIDS in Schools, promptly organized a boycott of the school. Anonymous bomb threats were made and then – the unimaginable. The Rays' home was burnt to the ground. The boys' uncle, Andy Ray, was in the house at the time of the fire and had to be treated for smoke inhalation. The Ray family has since moved to Sarasota, Florida, where the school board has a policy allowing children who are HIV positive to attend class.

One of the knock-on effects of all of the publicity surrounding these shocking events was to allow politicians from the extreme right a platform to vent their hatred of homosexuality, and to suggest that gay men and i.v. drug users should be segregated. Lyndon H. LaRouche Jr was already on his platform, and thumping the table hard. He had run in every presidential election since 1976, and was seeking the Democratic nomination in 1987. He supported California's Proposition 64, which demanded that infection with the virus should be treated as a notifiable disease. If passed, it would have meant that any infected person, even without AIDS symptoms, would be barred from all jobs involving contact with the public, and be subject to compulsory registration and enforced quarantine: in short, complete 'victimization' of people with HIV antibodies.

The idea was rejected, but it gives us pause for thought. If AIDS was declared an infectious disease, why was it *not* treated like other notifiable diseases, with isolation and periods of quarantine? Herein lies one of the fundamental contradictions in the AIDS story. The nightmare scenario of isolation units full of gay men, i.v. drug users and poor black and Hispanic Americans, those in fact who were in the high risk groups, combined with efforts to behave politically correctly towards gay men, made the authorities reluctant to classify AIDS as a notifiable disease. It would simply not have been acceptable to isolate such politically sensitive groups. This is yet further proof of how firmly embedded HIV and AIDS had remained within the high risk groups. Fear springs from ignorance, and those responsible for whipping up plague terror have made sure that no question marks remained in the air – the tyranny of their pseudo-scientific absolutism has left behind it a trail of horror. It is the individual tragedies, the waste of lives, that linger in one's mind. In January 1990, the *Sun* reported the suicide of hospital painter Arthur Rhodes after pricking his finger when catching a box of used hypodermics he knocked off a window ledge. 'Arthur, married with a 19-year-old son was "torn apart" by the worry,' writes Martyn Sharpe. 'Finally, he fixed a hosepipe to the exhaust of his new Toyota and died from carbon monoxide poisoning in the driveway of his parents' bungalow in Salkstone, Barnsley, Yorkshire.'[21]

The *Guardian*, 17 August 1989: '"AIDS" suicide'. 'A Greek policeman, George Ziogas, aged 25, shot himself because he believed he had AIDS, police said yesterday. His tests proved negative.' In London in 1994, a member of the Ugandan community told me that when a Ugandan man, living in London with his wife and two children, was told he was HIV positive, he became convinced his wife had infected him. He went home and killed his wife and his children. Nobody told that man that if you have had malaria you can develop 'sticky' cells that can show a false-positive result in an HIV test. Nobody told that man that being positive is not a death sentence. On the contrary, the HIV = AIDS = death mantra was only too audible even to the most caring doctor's ears. There are countless other stories. Young people in the prime of life, terrorized, committing suicide to relieve themselves of that intolerable death sentence.

In the Dominican Republic, in the village of Camu near the huge tourist complex of Puerto Plata, Hector Severino walks – barely walks – on one crutch. His left leg is totally twisted and deformed. He had a motorcycle accident. In hospital he was tested for HIV and found to be positive. The surgeon would not operate on his leg for fear of catching HIV so he was sent home to wait for his death. 'I was so unhappy, I lay on my bed and wept every day, and my wife wept with me,' he remembers. Severino's young wife became so terrified, she drank a whole bottle of bleach and took a month to die in agony. The story as it was told around the community was that the wife had been infected by her husband and died of AIDS. Today, the bereaved husband is in perfect health – but he can't walk. Having lost his job in the hotel industry, he is now too poor even to travel to see a doctor. A London-based AIDS charity offered £300 towards the cost of crutches, and further opinions on surgery for his leg.[22] Severino decided to use some of the funds to go into the nearby town of Puerto Plata to be retested for HIV. The test was negative. That was in 1995. A further test in 1996 proved negative as well. In 1997 Severino continued in excellent health. He had lost his job, his wife and the use of his leg. He had become isolated from his own community, he had thought he was going to die, and all because of an infernal HIV test that meant nothing in the first place.

The Epidemic Intelligence Service (EIS): Fanning the Flames of Plague Terror

It was the USA that took the lead in propagating the virus/AIDS hypothesis and it was a country with a built-in mechanism well prepared to do so. An organization called the Epidemic Intelligence Service (EIS) was formed at the Centers for Disease Control in 1951 under Alexander Langmuir. The EIS unit was originally composed of 23 young medical or public health graduates who, after a period of fieldwork and hospital training, would be free to pursue any career they desired on the assumption that their loyalties would remain with the CDC and that they would permanently act as its eyes and ears. Duesberg and Ellison have carefully documented this part of America's history:

The focus of this elite unit on activism rather than research was expressed in its symbol – a pair of shoe soles worn through with holes. As one former CDC consultant put it to us, epidemiologists have long referred to the service as the 'medical CIA'. Every summer since 1951 a new class of carefully-chosen EIS recruits has been trained, some classes exceeding one hundred people in size. Although a complete list of EIS officers and alumni is available, its members rarely advertise their affiliation. Over the last four decades, the CDC has quietly placed 2000 EIS trainees in key positions throughout the country and the world.[23]

Many members of this network are employed by the CDC itself, or by the federal government in different agencies. Some have become doctors and others work for international organizations like the WHO and in health departments of foreign governments. A few have moved into journalism and hold key positions in the US media. Lawrence Altman, for example, has been medical correspondent for the *New York Times* since 1969 and has maintained a high profile as supporter of the virus/AIDS hypothesis. EIS member Bruce Dan worked as medical correspondent for ABC News and then became senior editor of the prestigious *Journal of the American Medical Association.* 'Not only do they [EIS members] constitute an informal surveillance network,' say Duesberg and Ellison:

but they can even act as unrecognized advocates for the CDC viewpoint, whether as media journalists or as prominent physicians. . . . The CDC has exploited public trust by transforming flus and other minor epidemics into monstrous crises, and by manufacturing contagious plagues out of non-infectious medical conditions. Whereas the virus hunters at the NIH and academia have made themselves appear useful by blaming harmless or even non-existent viruses as culprits in well-established diseases, the CDC and its EIS infrastructure have possessed the resources needed to exaggerate or even fabricate the epidemics themselves. They have pushed the science establishment into action before anyone could raise questions, magnifying biomedical disasters beyond the wildest excesses of decades past.[24]

Duesberg and Ellison proceed to list a devastating catalogue of public health flops which involved the CDC and EIS: the Salk polio vaccine which led to hundreds of vaccine-induced polio cases; the panic whipped up about the 1957 Asian flu epidemic; the hype surrounding the sale of flu vaccines and the wild goose chases behind disease 'clusters' like the leukaemia clusters that the CDC always regarded as potential starting points for a contagious disease epidemic. The disastrous efforts to forestall a predicted swine flu epidemic led to plans for the most aggressive emergency immunization programme in history. But then it was discovered that in early testing, the vaccine produced side effects in 20 to 40 per cent of inoculated people. However, millions of people received the vaccine and soon there were reports of hundreds of cases of Guillain-Barré syndrome (paralysis) and 74 deaths from vaccine side effects.

The next fiasco was Legionnaire's disease, when some elderly members of the American Legion developed pneumonia and died after their annual reunion bash. Was this swine flu or a new contagious threat to the world? The EIS old boy network sprang into action and none other than Lawrence Altman of the *New York Times* was sent to cover the story. Nationwide hysteria developed and a CDC enquiry was set up. Nothing was found. 'The cavalier treatment and the one-track focus on infectious microbes,' write Duesberg and Ellison, 'so enraged New York Congressman John Murphy that he held hearings on Legionnaire's disease in 1976. Calling CDC officials to testify, Murphy humiliated the agency for not having found the epidemic's cause, and for ignoring the possibility of *non-contagious or toxic causes* [emphasis added].'[25] To save its hide, the CDC identified a harmless bacterium that inhabits soil, as well as plumbing in most buildings, and took credit for brilliantly discovering the cause of 'Legionnaire's disease'.

With the benefit of hindsight, it is astonishing that no one bothered to point out that no member of the hotel staff or indeed any women contracted the same illness, although they too were presumably breathing the same air. After the double fiascos of swine flu and Legionnaire's disease, the CDC was in the doldrums. The War on Cancer was also dragging on with no tangible results for the NIH. Both the CDC and the NIH needed a new challenge – a new plague. AIDS was their salvation.

That challenge came when Michael Gottlieb, a researcher at the University of California, Los Angeles, who was studying the immune system, found the first of the now famous cluster of young men with Kaposi's sarcoma, pneumocystis carinii pneumonia (PCP) and, of greatest interest to Gottlieb in terms of his research, all with a very low T-cell count – the white blood cells that participate in the immune system. It was not easy to find that cluster though. Gottlieb put out requests to be informed of further similar cases, and found two more. By April 1981, he decided he had a hot new syndrome on his hands and telephoned the Los Angeles public health department to ask for data on similar patients. There he spoke to Wayne Shandera, an active EIS officer, who found another case. They had found a pattern at last. All five men in the first 'cluster' were active homosexuals, and all used poppers, the amyl nitrite inhalant used to enhance sexual pleasure. Their condition was initially described as GRID – gay related immune deficiency.

James Curran at the CDC was contacted, and he hurried into print, calling the information 'hot stuff'. New cases emerged. Curran and his associates allowed only two alternative hypotheses on the agenda. Either this syndrome was caused by a single 'bad' batch of 'poppers' or it was contagious. No 'bad' batch of poppers was found so, based precariously on the notoriously unreliable 'cluster' model, they decided the syndrome had to be contagious. But what was the infectious agent? The wheels of the CDC began to turn faster. They called the syndrome 'Acquired Immune Deficiency Syndrome' (AIDS) and mobilized politicians and the press into declaring the dangers of this new epidemic.

One of the earliest converts was Dr Anthony Fauci at the National Institute of Allergy and Infectious Diseases (NIAID). He was to become one of the most ardent supporters of the CDC's view that AIDS was an infectious disease. Donald Francis of the CDC, who had worked with members of the virus-hunting Bob Club in the past, then linked the syndrome with feline leukaemia and decided AIDS had to be caused by a retrovirus. The new syndrome was declared contagious with a long latent period between infection and disease. 'This decision', write Duesberg and Ellyson, 'had no basis in any scientific evidence, but was destined to shape scientific thinking for years to come.'[26]

Within a year the entire world knew about AIDS and believed it to be infectious. Hundreds of millions and then thousands of millions of dollars began flowing into the NIH, the National Cancer Institute and other biomedical institutions. The virus hunters had finally reached the mother node. Robert Gallo was ready to pick up the baton and linked his leukaemia virus HTLV-I to a further variant, HTLV-III and thence to AIDS. The fateful press conference was held announcing HIV as the 'probable' cause of AIDS. And on that same day Gallo filed his US patent application for the HIV antibody test.

A hypothesis becomes doctrine when the majority of the scientific establishment accepts it. The well-oiled wheels of the CDC and EIS plague terror propaganda machinery made sure this happened. All research funding was funnelled into HIV, and any branches of AIDS research that were not virus-based were lopped off. Scientists need money for their research and every effort was made to lobby politicians for federal funding. Politicians need facts and statistics to justify their allocation of funds. These were made available with ever-increasing projections of a full-blown worldwide AIDS pandemic.

Fear of Heterosexual Spread

The UK lagged behind events in the USA. However, in November 1986 the Department of Health and Social Security decided to attack the presumed heterosexual spread of AIDS. Whole-page advertisements were taken out in the national newspapers. The *Guardian* on 28 November 1986 had this message across one page, 'AIDS IS NOT PREJUDICED. IT CAN KILL ANYONE. It's true more men than women have AIDS. But this does not mean it is a homosexual disease. It isn't. . . . . At the moment the infection is mainly confined to relatively small groups of people in this country. But the virus is spreading.' The actual figure for non-risk heterosexual spread in 1986 was under ten. In August 1987, the figures for AIDS deaths, non-risk (that means not infected abroad or not the child of an HIV positive parent) was only eight (three men and five women) out of a total of 192.

In September 1987, the UK Institute of Actuaries announced that there could be 57,000 cases of AIDS by 1999 if sexual habits did not change. The Institute had drawn up six different projections of the number of deaths from AIDS to the year 2012. Even the most conservative put deaths at more than 14,000 a year by the late 1990s.[27] (As of September 1996 the cumulative figure for AIDS deaths in the UK was 9447.) Propelled into action by all these public announcements, and by the January 1988 London Declaration in which international experts predicted a pandemic, the government launched a massive £20 million advertising campaign directed at the heterosexual community, involving house-to-house leafleting and a now infamous 40-second television commercial. The commercial's doom-laden scenario will go down in history as one of the most gruesome examples of official scaremongering. It opens with a mountain being sand-blasted for granite. Then an engraver's hand appears, chiselling out the letters AIDS on a granite tombstone. The tombstone swivels into an upright position in time for funereal lilies to fall on top together with a pamphlet, while the commentary says 'Don't die of ignorance.'

Then, in October 1988 the official government Cox Committee, which was advising the then Health Minister David Mellor, reported its predictions. These were set within wide limits and predicted between 1590 and 15,440 new cases per year to give a cumulative total of 8000 to 34,077 cases by the end of 1992. None of this happened. By the beginning of 1990 there was a cumulative total (since 1982) of 2800 registered AIDS cases (142 allegedly from heterosexual contact) and by 1992 a total of 6929 cases. The Cox Committee had estimated a mean figure of 17,125 (8000–34,077) – an overestimate of 147 per cent.

David Mellor a few years later conceded that too much public money had been spent on AIDS awareness campaigns directed at hetero-sexuals, but claimed he had felt pressured because of the alarming predictions of spread the committee had come up with. He had, he felt, been sorely ill-advised and would be prepared to say so in any future documentary we might be making.[28] During this period, Professor Gordon Stewart had been making strong efforts to get an article printed in which he based his predictions for AIDS on risk behaviour rather than the sexually infectious hypothesis. He maintained that even if Duesberg's arguments on HIV were laid aside, the epidemiological evidence did not support the idea that HIV was a sufficient cause of AIDS. Stewart is an eminent scientist and epidemi-ologist, famous for his work cleaning up early penicillin to get rid of allergenic residues, and developing the new penicillins. For many years he was Professor of Public Health at Glasgow University.

Stewart wrote to the MRC and to the Department of Health suggest-ing that the predictions were dangerously exaggerated when compared with trends since 1982. They did not respond. He then wrote to the

Royal Society, which expressed interest initially but held on to Stewart's paper until 1994 when it finally rejected it. Communications with *Nature*, the *British Medical Journal*, the *New England Journal of Medicine* and other journals were also rejected until the *Lancet* finally published a short letter from Stewart in 1993, accompanied by a cautious editorial comment.[29]

Looking back on his figures, which strongly criticized the Cox Committee's position (presented by various invited experts at the Royal Society's symposium in 1989), we find that Stewart was extraordinarily accurate. His predictions made in 1989 (which he had conveyed early in 1990 to the MRC and to the Royal Society) of 1254 cases in the UK in 1991 could not have been closer. The actual total of registered cases was 1275. Stewart's overall predictions for the decade 1982–92 were also extremely close. He predicted 6540 cases and the actual total was 6929.[30] Remember that Cox had quoted 12,750 or more for planning in this period.

Professor Stewart had been one of our scientific advisers through many of our science and medical programmes for television. We were in close touch with him when he made his predictions in 1989 and read all his correspondence with the different science journal editors. He was deeply frustrated. He was the only senior public health expert who offered a learned and detailed critique of the government's position, and not a single medical body or journal would give him an inch of space.

He says, 'The blank refusal of all the main medical societies and colleges, and nearly all the journals, to face the facts about AIDS is scandalous, and is probably the chief reason for the failure to develop a rational strategy to prevent a continuation of spread in the main risk groups and Third World countries.'[31] Stewart also says:

Apart from the accuracy (and mathematical simplicity of) my predictions, the main implications are (1) that the hypothesis that HIV is the necessary and sufficient cause of AIDS is not supported on epidemiological grounds; (2) that AIDS is not spreading except in groups engaging in or subjected to high risk behaviour; and (3) that there is no evidence in the USA, UK and northern Europe at least of any appreciable spread by heterosexual transmission or by vertical transmission to infants except from mothers in high risk groups.[32]

Stewart's projections for this period have been analysed by statistician Barrie Craven Ph.D., of the University of Northumbria. Together with other data from official sources, Craven has shown the absurdity of the pattern of expenditure on AIDS prevention across the world. He has also highlighted the questionable estimates for the spread of AIDS in Third World countries and pointed to the implications of his findings on future expenditure on AIDS. However, the censorship surrounding anyone challenging HIV meant that Stewart's views were completely ignored by the establishment.

A few, very few, journalists did raise criticisms of inflated figures for the spread of AIDS, among them James Le Fanu who pointed out that David Mellor had decided to take the highest possible figures from the Cox Committee and publicly announced that there could be as many as 30,000 cases of AIDS by 1992.[33] In subsequent articles, he attacked the way the threat of a heterosexual AIDS epidemic had been exaggerated. He described the way routine testing of pregnant women for HIV in inner London had reported a 'fourfold rise' in positive results. When he looked at the actual figures, they involved 18 out of 26,000 women tested in 1989, which rose to 32 out of 24,000 women the following year. 'So the fourfold increase actually represents an extra 14 cases,' he wrote. 'Quite frankly, it makes me sick.'[34]

Victoria Macdonald also made a swingeing attack on the government's 1989 advertising campaign aimed at heterosexuals, highlighting Lord Kilbracken's view that it was alarmist, wasteful and insane. Kilbracken, a member of the parliamentary group set up to look at the AIDS issue had released government statistics for June 1989 which stated that of the 2372 cases of full-blown AIDS in the UK, only one was known to be infected outside the high risk groups. Macdonald's article describes how the campaigns orchestrated by the Health Education Authority had themselves already run into trouble. It was rumoured that Margaret Thatcher had vetoed one slogan saying 'condoms are hip'. What eventually appeared was a picture of a beautiful woman bearing the caption, 'How will this young woman look in ten years if she has AIDS?' In a following page an identical picture of the young woman appeared, suggesting that HIV has a long incubation period and appearances can be deceptive.

At the time the advertisement appeared the former president of the Royal College of Surgeons, Sir Reginald Murley, suggested to Mrs Thatcher that the caption should have read: 'Fortunately this young woman is unlikely to develop AIDS unless she becomes a drug addict or allows herself to be buggered.'[35]

Chapter 6

'The AIDS Catch'

The Dissident Censored

It was in this climate of fear and panic that we decided to make another programme about AIDS. I telephoned Peter Duesberg, and asked him if anything had changed since we made the last programme and whether he had had any doubts. He said, 'On the contrary I am more than ever convinced that HIV is not the cause of AIDS.' Later he called specifically to say, 'I do not believe AIDS is an infectious disease at all.' It was time for me to visit Duesberg in his own setting and see if we could take the AIDS debate a step further.

His laboratory is set among fir trees on top of the Berkeley campus hill with a breathtaking view of the Bay Bridge and San Francisco's skyscrapers across the water. It was raining when I arrived one weekend and the laboratory was empty. There are two laboratories, one each side of the corridor. His office is tucked away in the corner of the front laboratory. Pinned above his desk is a note saying, 'The only stupid questions are the ones not asked.' So I asked and asked.

Soon Bryan Ellison walked in, a young postdoctoral student who was to play a big part in the Duesberg story later on. Today he was visiting Peter for a chat. We sat on three laboratory stools drinking Chinese tea in paper cups for literally hours, while he and Peter discussed the AIDS situation and whether molecular biology had become so concentrated on looking further and further down the electron microscope that it had forgotten or did not know how to interpret what it saw.

The conversation with Duesberg was to continue at the local cafe and at his flat, occasionally interrupted by one of his three daughters

74

popping in for money for this or that. Married with three daughters, Duesberg was separated from his German wife Astrid, having left her in the big house on the hill behind Berkeley, while he moved into dingy lodgings in a rickety building on the edge of a motorway in Oakland. His flat was spartan and made one feel he was punishing himself for this self-imposed exile. He had few mod cons and a spoon stuck out of an ancient black and white TV set 'to make it work'. I noticed that his tiny hallway was blocked by a pile of papers, rising three feet off the ground. 'That' he said, 'is evidence of the battle I fought to get my AIDS paper published in the *Proceedings of the National Academy of Sciences*.'

After publication of his cancer research paper, Duesberg decided to write a review of the AIDS literature and turned to the journal of the exclusive National Academy, called *Proceedings of the National Academy of Sciences* (*PNAS*). Duesberg had been a member of the academy since 1986 for his achievements in virology, retrovirology and his discovery, along with his colleague Peter Vogt, of oncogenes. He had spent 16 hours a day seven days a week for six months researching and writing his 7500-word paper called 'HIV and AIDS: correlation but not causation'.[1] Normally, members of the academy expect to be able to publish their papers with a review from one experienced colleague who is not a coauthor. But things were different for Duesberg. I have a 50-page dossier of the correspondence exchanged between Duesberg and two of the *PNAS* editors, Maxine Singer and Igor Dawid, between June and September 1988.

The correspondence is a classic example of the way a ruling scientific orthodoxy can so easily stifle a challenge through the flawed process of anonymous peer review. Had it not been for Duesberg's colossal tenacity and the open-mindedness of editor Igor Dawid (who eventually did publish the paper), this major contribution to the understanding of AIDS would never have seen the light of day.

Peer Review and Suppressing Debate

To understand how a mistaken scientific orthodoxy like that of AIDS can become as entrenched as it has, one has to understand the process of peer review. When an editor of a scientific journal receives an article intended for publication, he shows it to one or more referees to ensure that it is good science. Editors choose their own referees who remain anonymous.

Not surprisingly, nearly everyone who might be considered suitable to review Duesberg's work was already heavily immersed in HIV-based research funding. So, Duesberg had countless attempts at publication turned down because of the peer review process. *Nature*'s editor, John Maddox (later Sir John), has repeatedly rejected Duesberg's work. Yet Maddox himself pointed out the iniquities of the peer review system to journalist Adrian Berry in his article on biology 'Death of a life science'.[2]

'The epoch-making paper by Francis Crick and James Watson,' wrote Berry, 'outlining the structure of DNA, which appeared in *Nature* in 1953, would "probably not be published today", Mr Maddox laments, because the referees, those anonymous "experts" to whom scientific journal editors refer manuscripts for approval, would have raised niggling questions the authors might not have been able to answer.' The article goes on to describe how excruciatingly boring the published data on biology have become with journals like *Nature* and others 'prone to filling pages with nucleotide sequences that resemble secret service cryptograms'. Maddox goes on to say (quite prophetically as it happens) that 'Future historians may think it odd that so much should have been learnt about molecules on which life depends while so little has been understood about their function or about life itself.'

In a further article called 'Arrogant scientists suppress new ideas',[3] Berry quotes Dr David Horrobin, editor of *Medical Hypotheses* and *Prostaglandins*. 'The system is breaking down,' says Horrobin.

The referees write things anonymously in their reports that they wouldn't dare write if they were required to add their signatures. About one third [of referees] are sound and sensible. Another third are accurate but annoyingly nit-picking, while the remaining third write such scurrilous and disreputable comments that their work is a disgrace. The result is that new ideas are being suppressed.

Proceedings of the National Academy of Sciences

Duesberg submitted his review article to the *PNAS* on 13 June 1988. It had already been critically read and recommended for publication by his colleagues, Professors Harry Rubin and G. Steven Martin. Despite this, the paper was rejected on 30 June 1988 by Maxine Singer who, on the last day in her post as chairperson of the *PNAS* editorial board, wrote to Duesberg saying: 'For a review article, I believe that a fresh collection of primary data or innovative analysis of older data constitute originality. Unfortunately, I do not see either of these attributes in your manuscript. . . . These considerations have led me to conclude that the *Proceedings* ought not to publish this manuscript.' If he wished to discuss this conclusion further, Duesberg should contact her successor, Dr Igor Dawid. On 14 July Duesberg wrote to Igor Dawid saying that he considered Singer's decision inappropriate, as both of his reviewers had considered the paper both original and the material very up-to-date. 'I believe that it is my right,' he wrote, 'as a member of the Academy involved in a serious scientific controversy on a subject of clinical relevance, to publish my views in the *Proceedings*. It would be against the spirit of academic freedom to close the *Proceedings* to such an important scientific cause.'[4] After much wrangling and further anonymous peer reviews, Duesberg finally got his paper published, but not without a monumental struggle, in February 1989[5]. It was followed by another in 1991 called 'AIDS epidemiology: inconsistencies with human immunodeficiency virus and with infectious disease'.[6]

I flew home determined to make another programme. The heat was on. Duesberg was being bombarded with telephone calls at his laboratory from all over the world. It was time to bring to the public's attention the arguments we had been able to follow through Duesberg, but which had been contained behind the closed doors of the scientific establishment. I drafted an outline for another programme, called it 'AIDS II' and sent it to Duesberg. He made his comments and then suddenly telephoned to say he had reached the point where he could see clearly why AIDS was not infectious and ran through his key arguments. I renamed the outline 'AIDS – Infectious or Not?' and sent it to David Lloyd.

Lloyd was keen to do another programme. After all, our first one had made history in that it was the first time ever that an independent company had won a coveted Royal Television Society award. He gave us a development budget and off we went on the research round. We set out to find evidence of the most glaring anomalies in the virus/AIDS hypothesis and to demand answers to questions surrounding these anomalies. For example:

- If HIV is supposed to be so lethal why, of the one million HIV positives in the USA, over a period of eight years, have only 1.5 per cent developed AIDS?
- Why is it mostly men who contract AIDS? (90 per cent in the USA.)
- If AIDS is infectious through HIV, why has AIDS remained confined to the risk groups (intravenous drug users and highly promiscuous homosexual men)?
- How is it possible to have AIDS without HIV and HIV without AIDS?

The Pause Between the Beat: Where the Truth Lies

Author Paul Scott once said, after writing the *Raj Quartet*, that it is in 'the pause between the beat of history' that the truth really lies, and this is what we set out to find.

One of our first tasks was to meet Professor Luc Montagnier face to face. We waited for him sitting on a bench outside his laboratory at the Pasteur Institute in Paris. He did not see us as he approached, wrapped in thought and in a big black overcoat flapping around his calves. A small rounded man with a baby face, he looked like a man reluctantly catapulted to fame. His fame was not without controversy. His first paper on the AIDS virus had been signed by five authors, including his co-workers Drs Françoise Barre-Sinoussi and Claude Chermann. Both became bitterly disaffected, feeling that they were deprived of the HIV laurels and of returns from the test patent.

It is interesting now to reread the carefully worded press release given to us by the Pasteur Institute on our visit.

'The AIDS Catch'

In 1983, researches at the Viral Oncology Unit led by Professor Luc Montagnier have played a major role in the isolation and characterization of the AIDS *virus, Human Immunodeficiency Virus or* HIV, *in collaboration with clinicians and immunologists of several hospitals in Paris. In less than two years, the virus was molecularly analysed and its genetic make up was unravelled by a team of five young molecular biologists. . . . Independently, US researchers made similar findings.*

Until our meeting with Montagnier that day in early March 1990, the world had been led to believe that if you caught HIV it would kill you willy nilly. Yet, we were about to hear some earth shattering news that the very scientist who discovered HIV was now back-pedalling on the virus's ability to be the sole cause of AIDS. Montagnier had been working on the theory that certain cofactors might be necessary to trigger HIV. He had found something he described as mycoplasmas that he felt combined with HIV to cause AIDS.

Montagnier greeted Michael Verney-Elliott and me warmly in his office and proceeded to explain his position. I have series of quotes from our meeting:

We should not have said in the first place that HIV *might explain everything. If that were the case we should find no disease at all by now.*

HIV *by itself is not a very dangerous virus. But it has to be there. Without it nothing can happen.*

I always took a cautious view on the virus and from Cold Spring Harbor in 1983 I said we should be looking for other things.

I have been looking for co-factors since 1983. I am working on some microbial agents as possible co-factors.

Montagnier told us he was very enthusiastic about his mycoplasma work. I suggested that if he was *speculating* about possible different co-factors, then surely he must be *speculative* about HIV? He said he was really talking about co-agents. What was the difference, I asked? He said 'co-agents have the same importance and with co-factors there's one primary agent.' Then he waved his hands and said, 'It's all semantics really.' Duesberg's view on co-factors is that when they are invoked, they are the sign of a bankrupt hypothesis, because how can you tell which is the real cause of the disease?

We had noticed how the word 'co-factors' had begun to creep into the language of the orthodoxy – something Duesberg had already predicted would happen. He said:

Once you have an establishment that has made a mistake, but got into a position of power for it, they will hardly resign because it's very comfortable to be there on top. It's a nice place to be. Now, when you see it's not working, you have two choices. Either you say it's wrong or you say it's working but not the way we initially thought. It's somewhat more complicated. And the classic escape in science is to say it [HIV] is not sufficient to cause the disease, which is what they've been saying from the beginning. They now say we need something else.

They now say it's not sufficient, but it is still necessary. If it weren't necessary, of course, they would have to resign and would have to revise prevention and therapy. . . . To say it's necessary means they stay in business and it gives them plenty of time to adjust their hypothesis. But by doing this you question your primary claim directly, because if you don't know what else causes it you can't know whether HIV plays a role in it. Until you know the other element and show that it needs HIV to cause something – like the mycoplasma claim – you have to take the mycoplasma and show that it needs HIV to cause AIDS, or whatever effect it might have. Until this is done you have no proof whatsoever that HIV plays a role in it.[7]

Montagnier was keen that we include his mycoplasma theory in our film and we agreed to do so. As it happened, Montagnier's mycoplasma theory went down like a lead balloon at the subsequent San Francisco International AIDS conference. An audience of HIV-can-do-it-alone fanatics heckled, hissed and booed him, which led him to leave the conference early in a huff.

As we travelled back to London, Michael and I felt that Montagnier was finding himself in a situation where he was having serious doubts about the role of HIV but could hardly let it go altogether. HIV test kit royalties were providing a steady 5 per cent of the Pasteur Institute's funding. Nonetheless, it seemed to us that his scientific nouse was making him try to find a way out of blaming only HIV for AIDS.

The AIDS Catch:
Exposing the Myths around HIV and AIDS

Our first port of call was Paris to record the interview with Montagnier based on our previous discussions. Montagnier's performance on film was just as strong as for our research interview. Asked whether he had always believed that HIV on its own could cause AIDS, his response reverberated around the world:

At first, yes, we thought we had the best candidate for this virus to be the cause of AIDS. But after a while – even from the beginning actually – we thought maybe for the activation of that virus in cells we had to – we need some co-factors. . . . So I would agree that HIV by itself, or some strains of HIV are not sufficient to induce AIDS.[8]

This statement confirmed Montagnier's position from the very beginning. He had never been as categorical as Gallo in pointing the finger at HIV as the sole (sufficient) cause of AIDS. Now he was publicly voicing his doubts and drawing in the co-factor theory – that HIV needed other factors to trigger it into producing harmful effects.

In New York we paid an important visit to Dr Joe Sonnabend's surgery. As one of the earliest 'AIDS dissidents', in 1984 he had published a broadsheet called *AIDS Research*. It was too dangerous for the orthodoxy, was quickly muzzled, lost its funding and was taken over by Burroughs Wellcome as an information sheet about (predictably) the latest AIDS drug therapies. Sonnabend, an immensely caring doctor, worked from a small dingy surgery in Manhattan, looking after the scores of young gay men who came to him with a string of different infections and reinfections. It was he who inspired Michael Callen and Richard Berkowitz to examine the lifestyle factors that could be at the root of the severe immune suppression young gay men were experiencing.[9]

Sonnabend looked as though he were neglecting himself, with dandruff collecting on his black jacket which was several sizes too small for him. He had grown despondent. No one was prepared to fund any meaningful research into the syndrome that was affecting his patients. Sonnabend had never been convinced by HIV. His view was that the immune-suppression described as AIDS was brought on by multiple factors involving risk behaviour that included infectious components. He told us: 'I would believe that the infectious components are a variety of common or well-known infections including virus infections such as cytomegalovirus infection (a type of herpes), sexually transmitted diseases, such as syphilis and a variety of common infections which are known to have immune suppressive components.'[10]

Author and AIDS chronicler John Lauritsen received us in his little flat in Greenwich Village. He focused his attention on toxicity rather than infectivity as the cause of immune suppression in AIDS, blaming the harmful effects of recreational drugs like poppers and the damage done by the AIDS drug AZT (both of which we will deal with in more detail separately). Another revealing episode occurred when we interviewed Dr Alvin Friedman-Kein at New York University. A specialist in Kaposi's sarcoma that was once seen as the cornerstone of the AIDS diagnosis, now, curiously, Friedman-Kein was finding cases of KS in people without HIV. Could this be AIDS without HIV? Michael asked him. Unlikely, said Friedman-Kein, because there was no evidence of immune suppression in these men. They simply had the well-documented non-invasive form of KS that had been described in medical literature since the last century.

However, Friedman-Kein put us in touch with one of his KS patients who was HIV negative. We met Alan outside New York University Hospital and we were shocked by his appearance. Here was a man who, according to Friedman-Kein had no evidence of immune suppression and was supposed to be perfectly well except for KS, yet standing before us was a man with all the appearance of AIDS. His shirt collar drooped loosely around his pathetically thin neck. His skin had that waxen yellow look. It stretched across his face like a mask. His baggy trousers hid the thinnest legs, which could hardly carry him as he ambled towards us like an old man. Yes, he had lost a hell of a lot of weight. Yes, he had been highly promiscuous both with men and women. Yes, he had taken a hell of a lot of poppers and other drugs. So this was a patient Friedman-Kein said couldn't possibly have AIDS because he had no HIV?

During our filmed interview with Friedman-Kein, Michael challenged him saying, 'I'm a little confused. You said earlier that in the case of these HIV negative men, they have no other symptoms and they have no immune suppression, so why have they got Kaposi's sarcoma if it's an opportunistic disease?' Friedman-Kein couldn't really answer this. He murmured something about 'another transmissible agent' possibly causing KS. He then said that the CDC and other scientists around the country were reconsidering the definition of AIDS 'to perhaps change the definition not to include Kaposis's sarcoma as a definitive diagnosis'.[11]

It was an altogether unconvincing performance and supported Duesberg's point that whenever AIDS-defining diseases are found without HIV, the patients are diagnosed as having that specific condition, but not AIDS. Therefore, by definition, all cases like Alan's are lost to AIDS statistics. Because they are HIV negative, they are not followed up. They don't come back for a second test and, as health researcher Michelle Cochrane discovered in San Francisco, without a second seronegative test, these cases are lost to statistics. This is why there are so few registered cases of AIDS without HIV.

Professor Robert Root-Bernstein came to our rescue on the KS matter. He had been studying the history of KS and believed that KS itself, without HIV can produce an irreversible AIDS-type condition. When we interviewed him later in San Francisco, he said:

The existence of Kaposi's sarcoma patients who are HIV negative suggests to me that there are causes of AIDS other than HIV. In fact, I've just completed a study of Kaposi's sarcoma that goes back to the very first paper ever published on the subject by Maurice Kaposi in 1872 and it shows that in fact there are hundreds of Kaposi's sarcoma patients matching the CDC definition of AIDS over a century. These patients are not elderly men, these are teenage boys, they are young men in their 20s and 30s, they are often described as being previously healthy.[12]

In April 1990, the *Lancet* published a letter from Root-Bernstein in which he describes specific cases of young men, including a five-year-old boy who died of KS within a year in the 1880s. They all had penile lesions and respiratory failure accompanying high fever and possibly pneumonia. The letter merits quoting at length.

There was no test for HIV until 1984 but if we accept that HIV is a new retrovirus that entered North America and Europe in the past two or three decades, then all of the cases listed above must have been HIV free. If so, several hypotheses must be entertained – that AIDS is not new; that HIV is only one of several possible causes of AIDS; or that HIV is itself a new, opportunistic infection that takes advantage of previously immunosuppressed individuals. If, however, one argues that KS in otherwise healthy young men is always associated with HIV, these historical cases would indicate that HIV is not a new disease agent, and it would follow that AIDS is not a new disease and that the current epidemic is due not to the introduction of a new virus but to changes in lifestyle creating a population of susceptible individuals and/or extending modes of transmission. The existence of HIV-free AIDS cases requires us to re-evaluate the theory that AIDS is a new disease and that HIV is the necessary and sufficient cause.[13]

Meeting Root-Bernstein was exciting. Awarded the coveted MacArthur Prize Fellowship – a five-year 'genius' award – he had later produced an excellent paper called 'Do we know the cause(s) of AIDS?' which he had sent to Duesberg to look through. In it Root-Bernstein argued that 'the conclusion that HIV is the sole cause of immunosuppression in AIDS and the sole factor differentiating AIDS patients from non-AIDS patients, cannot be maintained.'[14]

Root-Bernstein had never met Duesberg, so Channel 4 agreed to fly him from a conference in Florida to Berkeley for our interview. There, Peter had arranged for him to give a seminar. But incredibly, when Duesberg requested the use of a lecture hall in the centre of the campus he was told the subject was too dangerous and controversial to be in such a public place, so we all had to be bused to a remote lecture hall at the top of a hill (ironically, where the atom bomb had been developed).

Root-Bernstein gave his talk, which was largely hostile to the virus/ AIDS hypothesis, although there were points of disagreement between him and Duesberg. Duesberg gave him a pretty rough grilling during question time. Bryan Ellison was furious. 'Why do you have to attack one of our few supporters like that?' he said. 'You have to attack your friends intellectually just as strongly as you attack your enemies,' said Duesberg. The moral high ground on the HIV debate was captured with great eloquence by Professor Walter Gilbert, a most distinguished US scientists and Nobel prize winner, a wise man who, unlike many of his over-hasty colleagues, had never attached himself publicly to the HIV hypothesis and was therefore able to voice some serious doubts about the science surrounding it. He was concerned at the way the media and parts of the scientific community had blown up the virus as the cause of AIDS:

because it is more convenient to have a neat explanation. The community as a whole doesn't listen patiently to critics who adopt alternative viewpoints, although the great lesson of history is that knowledge develops through the conflict of viewpoints. If you have simply a consensus, it generally stultifies. It fails to see the problems of that consensus and it depends on the existence of critics to break up that iceberg and permit knowledge to develop. This is in fact one of the underpinnings of democratic theory. It's one of the basic reasons why we believe in notions of free speech and it's one of the great forces in terms of intellectual development.[15]

One of the most revealing and yet intriguing anomalies in the AIDS story awaited us in St Petersburgh, Florida. We met Ron Webeck at his parents' comfortable home by the waterside. He had become famous as 'the man who lost HIV'. He decided to tell us his story.

Ron admitted to us that he had led a self-destructive lifestyle. He had lived in the gay fast lane, working as a waiter on the East Coast and in Europe. He had had many different sexual partners, took poppers, marijuana, and abused alcohol. In 1985 he was working as a waiter in Cape Cod, when he began to get headaches and a pain in his neck and back. He then found he couldn't add up his clients' bills properly, developed tunnel vision and began to limp badly. He was rushed to hospital where they found HIV and an AIDS related brain condition called PML (progressive multifocal leukoencephalopathy) allegedly caused by the so-called JC virus. He was very ill for six months and even signed a 'Do Not Resuscitate' order.

After a while he asked the doctors to send him home because he thought he was going to die and wanted to die at home. However, once home, he got better and better and he decided to fight for his life. 'The first thing I did was I asked my parents to get me a walker so I could maybe teach myself to walk again, as the doctors never really thought I would walk. They never bothered to rehabilitate me so I rehabilitated myself.'[16] He said the worst thing was visiting the local swimming pool, because people who had heard about him got out of the water when he went in. Then, in 1989, when Ron went back for tests at the NIH, to their astonishment, the doctors could find no trace of HIV, either in his blood or his spinal column, and the JC virus had disappeared as well. A second batch of test confirmed these findings, and Ron Webeck's case was reported in *Annals of Internal Medicine*.[17]

When we met up with Ron he looked very well and we filmed him going for a swim in the sea. However, even though he was HIV negative, his doctors had persuaded him to take AZT. Michael tried to point out the dangers of this therapy, but Ron continued to take it. He suffered a further series of strokes and two years later he was dead. There was still no sign of HIV. Had he been wise to continue with his AZT therapy? The toxic effects of AZT will be described in detail in a separate chapter below.

In San Francisco we were to interview Dr Andrew Moss, an English epidemiologist working at San Francisco General Hospital, which was the centre for AIDS treatment. Moss looked like a man who had put on a lot of weight recently and was not happy about it. He had an air of tolerant superiority about him when we told him we were interviewing Duesberg and other critics of the HIV hypothesis. Although he himself was committed to the virus/AIDS hypothesis and had voiced strong criticism of Duesberg, he had also been critical of the way in which predictions for the spread of AIDS had been made. He had no doubt that AIDS would spread into the heterosexual community and was confident that anyone who was HIV positive would progress to AIDS within nine and a half years.

I think most official predictions about the spread of AIDS have been consistently wrong in this country, and in Britain and in the world, and I think there are two reasons for that. One is a lot of very bad science was done, and the other is the political pressures to have high numbers. All administrative numbers are political. And that usually inflates from the opposite direction, and I think it's been hard for people to back away from their high numbers.[18]

Head of Stanley Laboratory at Berkeley and colleague of Peter Duesberg, Professor Harry Rubin had always lent a sympathetic ear, supporting Duesberg against his critics and defending his right to challenge the orthodoxy. Looking like a wise Jewish elder with a twinkle in his eye he said, 'Peter has been called all sorts of names and he's been labelled crazy . . . but they've been *ad hominem* attacks rather than thorough scientific, unprejudiced analyses of what he has to say. So by bucking the system and doing it with his characteristic flair he has aroused a lot of antagonism.'[19] Was it a good thing for scientists to buck the system and question, asked Michael? 'Well, I think it's a good thing for society in general and it's good for science. It's not too healthy for the scientists who do it. It affects recognition, grants, getting graduate students, all the things that go with scientific achievement.'[20]

And finally, on to Duesberg himself. We had to make sure that he gave of his best. He is a hopelessly fidgety interviewee, mischievously leaning out of camera frame every now and then to take a drink of water out of a plastic cup, and interrupting the interviewee with a succession of quips. All very well, but, we needed weighty delivery on this sombre subject. So we whipped him into shape and he certainly did deliver, interrupted only by the incessant chiming of the campus campanile clock.

Duesberg put the view that HIV can do very little in its human host, that it becomes neutralized by the immune system a couple of weeks or months after the infection and then does nothing more. He said that

AIDS was not spreading like a sexually transmitted disease should, but had remained within certain risk groups, namely intravenous drug users and a small percentage of male homosexuals. He explained how AIDS did not comply with Robert Koch's postulates (the conditions by which an infectious disease can be identified and distinguished from a toxic reaction). He explained how the goal posts for AIDS-defining diseases had been consistently revised by the Centers for Disease Control and how the latency period had been extended year by year. He also described his concern about the toxicity of AZT. Then he came on to the crux of his argument.

I believe AIDS is not, or cannot even be an infectious disease. An infectious disease, believe it or not, has a certain criteria to it. How it happens, when it happens. For example, if you get infected by a bug or by a virus, within weeks or months after contact or after that infection you will have symptoms of a disease. In HIV and AIDS, however, we are told you get sick ten years later, ten years after infection. That is not how viruses or bacteria work. They work fast or never. They are a very simple mechanism like a little clock that can do only one thing – go around the dial once and that takes 24 to 48 hours with a virus. There's no way that a virus could possibly slow down or wait a week or wait ten years. That is totally absurd.

AIDS, as it is thought of, is primarily a result of, I suspect, intoxication – Acquired Immune Deficiency – as the word actually says. In AIDS you acquire it by consuming drugs, and through malnutrition that is often typically linked to it. Once that has happened, once you are immune deficient, then you are open to many infections that are secondary or opportunistic as we say. That is not therefore an infectious disease, it is the result *of that.*

If the infectious hypothesis is proved to be wrong, asked Michael, at the end, what then? 'The implications would be very serious,' said Duesberg, 'very, very serious in fact. Millions of lives that could have been saved won't be saved if we work on an ungrounded or poorly grounded hypothesis. AIDS prevention, which is now entirely based on preventing contacts with infected people would take a totally different direction.'[21]

As we boarded the plane back to London, we knew then that we had a powerful programme on our hands. When we had gathered our thoughts and our evidence together we went back to David Lloyd. I said I really wanted to ride the horse this time and argue firmly from the dissident standpoint. David agreed, remembering that there had been hundreds of hours of television time devoted unchallenged to the orthodox view. 'As long as we signpost it,' he said. And we did. We said, 'This programme traces evidence that contradicts HIV as the cause of AIDS. We question whether AIDS is an infectious disease at all.'

AZT Toxicity: AIDS and the Weller Episode

David Lloyd wanted a section on AZT in our film. AZT is the drug that was initially prescribed to people with AIDS symptoms and post 1989 to people who were HIV positive with no symptoms of AIDS.

I shall be devoting a chapter to our AZT programme later on. But at the time of *The AIDS Catch* filming there was already considerable controversy about the drug's high toxicity. Many gay men had watched their partners with AIDS suffer appalling effects from the drug and then die. High doses of 1500 milligrams a day were being prescribed and patients were experiencing projectile vomiting, bone-marrow depletion needing blood transfusions, and unendurable headaches. The high dose regimen required strict compliance on a four-hourly basis, so people were given little pill containers with alarms in them to remind them to take their pills. The Royal Opera House at Covent Garden was often filled with the sound of insistent bleeping in the middle of the most heartrending arias.

Author John Lauritsen had already written exhaustively on the dangers of AZT, and Peter Duesberg had expressed grave concern at the way AZT was actually producing symptoms indistinguishable from the symptoms of AIDS. We decided to interview Professor Ian Weller who was coordinating the UK arm of a very big three-year Anglo-French AZT study called the Concorde trial. Its aim was to discover if AZT could delay the development of AIDS in people who were HIV positive but without symptoms of AIDS.

Weller gave us a very revealing interview. Obviously a man of conscience, as subsequent events would show, Weller looked worried. Having started out on the study with the best of intentions, he was now finding himself having to justify doling out a highly toxic drug to men who were essentially well, but not being able properly to identify whether they were suffering from a progression to AIDS or from the effects of the AZT itself. Under searching questioning from Michael, he said that the earlier US studies that had led to the licensing of AZT for asymptomatic patients had not been properly blinded. That is to say, doctors could tell who was on the drug and who was on the placebo (the dummy). This he thought could have led to bias in the trial's results. He admitted that the commonest side effect of AZT was its effect on bone marrow. It could lead to a lowered white blood cell count and anaemias which, if not monitored, could be serious enough for the patient to require blood transfusions.

He admitted that in some susceptible patients the bone marrow damage could be irreversible, but suggested that in these cases it could be 'more due to the virus affecting the bone marrow than the drug'. Weller said, 'With asymptomatic disease, it can be quite difficult to sort out what is due to the drug and what is due to the disease itself. It's as if you are looking, in a way, at the natural history of HIV infection behind a curtain of zidovudine (generic name for AZT). So it's difficult to differentiate between those two effects.'[22]

Weller acknowledged here that he could not differentiate between the effects of AZT and the effects of HIV infection. When Duesberg read the interview transcript, the crucial question he wanted to ask Weller was: What did Weller do when faced with these patients in his study who needed blood transfusions while on AZT therapy? Did he continue with AZT therapy, or did he stop it? His point being that if Weller did not know whether it was the virus or the drug that was doing the damage, by not stopping the drug, people could be actually dying because of the AZT therapy alone.

As the film came together, the first ever to confront the AIDS orthodoxy, there were so many major issues to tackle that less and less space remained for AZT. We decided to include only Duesberg and Lauritsen as critics. To try to embrace the complexities of the Concorde trial and some of Ian Weller's self-damning admissions seemed a little unfair. It would have been like setting him up as an Aunt Sally. So we did not include him. The words on AZT broadcast on film in *The AIDS Catch* were uncompromising:

DUESBERG: *The mechanism of action of AZT is embarrassingly clear and simple. It is a terminator of DNA synthesis. DNA is the basis for all life on this planet. It's the central molecule in every living cell.*

LAURITSEN: *Well, I have examined all of the major studies which are used to claim benefits for AZT. Without exception I would say these studies prove nothing. They have been in one respect or another incompetent and/ or dishonest, but I would maintain there is no scientifically credible evidence whatsoever that AZT has benefits to anybody under any circumstance.*

(to DUESBERG): *What do you think of the current trials looking into the long-term effects of AZT?*

DUESBERG: *'Well I think they will just show again that AZT is toxic. If you give less it will take longer to kill somebody with it ... and if you take more it goes faster.*[23]

The film's transmission date was 13 June 1990. Channel 4 held a press conference before it. Duesberg flew over for it and it was chaired by David Lloyd's deputy Karen Brown. (She later told me she had been completely taken aback by the fury expressed at the meeting.) There were many gay activists there. Cass Mann, of Positively Healthy, was very supportive, but others like Simon Watney angrily criticized the film. Watney made an emotional outburst about all the friends he knew who were dying of AIDS who would be ill-served by this film. Predictably, there was precious little discussion about the science behind the facts. When the film was broadcast, this time, far from a pool of silence, there was a mighty explosion.

Chapter 7
Fall Out

The Establishment Hits Back: Managing the Media

We had our production team gathering at my home on the night of transmission. Duesberg was still with us and some of his London friends from the old days of oncogene work joined us. As the programme ended, calls began to flood into Channel 4's duty office. That was just the beginning. Years later, the letters and articles that followed make astonishing reading. Every major medical organization, science journal and national newspaper (except the *Financial Times*) and every arm of the scientific establishment voiced its fury and vitriol. The rage focused on the fear that by questioning HIV we were encouraging promiscuity and unprotected sex among young people, who thus risked exposure to AIDS. Never did it occur to the critics that the premises of the HIV = AIDS = death might at least be worth questioning.

The MRC's Dr D. Rees fired off a letter to Sir George Russell, chairman of the Independent Broadcasting Authority. The MRC had involved millions of pounds of taxpayers' money in HIV research projects, many of them ongoing. Rees said, 'there is overwhelming scientific evidence that HIV infection is a necessary precondition for the development of AIDS. ... It is the gross irresponsibility of misleading the public by promulgating such views without balancing information which concerns me.' Rees said, the programme 'does grave disservice to public health. It is not an exaggeration to say that, should [the] *Dispatches* hypothesis be believed by viewers, lives will be put at risk.'[1]

We were asked by Channel 4 to draft a letter of reply to the MRC which ended, 'We take exception to your remark that "lives will be put at risk" by our programme. There is a far greater danger in resting complacently upon a consensus view which is unproven and has not succeeded in saving one life.' Next came the British Medical Association Foundation for AIDS letter to David Lloyd signed by its administrator, Hilary Curtis. It listed '14 major errors' in the film and said 'In putting forward a speculative notion that poly-drug misuse is the cause of AIDS, without supporting evidence, this programme may have significantly damaged the public health as well as causing distress to people living with AIDS and HIV'.[2] (Our programmes had been the only ray of hope anyone living with HIV had had in ten years!)

Virologist Jonathan Weber's piece for the *British Medical Journal* entitled 'Heresy and HIV', called it a 'misleading programme' and said, 'Duesberg makes great television but terrible public health, and I am grateful that he is restricted only to publicizing his ideas rather than putting them into action.'[3] A lead article in the *New Scientist* said, 'The cause of science on British Television took a step backwards last night with the transmission on Channel 4 of the documentary entitled *The AIDS Catch*.'[4] Julian Meldrum, a journalist writing for *Capital Gay*, wrote a particularly vicious attack on Duesberg. He said:

I have ploughed through many pages of Duesberg's rambling thoughts in search of any positive call or suggestion of research that could conceivably benefit people with AIDS. There are none. On the contrary, he seems most concerned that excessive amounts of money are being spent on 'irrelevant' research into a virus and disease that will, in his view, continue to be confined to gay men and drug users. I think he now deserves nothing but contempt.[5]

The intellectual level of some of our critics and their more puerile remarks must go on record. In a British Medical Association (BMA) newsletter, entitled 'Dangerous Dispatches' one Hal Satterthwaite, staff nurse at the ROMA Project that cares for AIDS patients, wrote:

The programme needs to be watched four or five times before it can be believed that it is actually saying some of these things. It is not a process that is recommended. At least one person taking notes from the pro-

gramme (a bit like taking notes from someone extremely drunk – quite difficult and very frustrating) has been seen foaming at the mouth.[6]

There were some glimmers of approval. Professor Roy Wilkie, at Strathclyde University, phoned in after the programme expressing interest and approval. Professor P. D. Wall, a developmental biologist at the Middlesex School of Medicine wrote to the *Independent* saying:

I detect excessive reaction in the cries of 'irresponsibility' directed at Channel 4 and the participants in the AIDS programme. ... Both [sides] insist that we should all avoid 'like the plague' any action that will insert foreign mucky protein into the bloodstream. There is a genuine difference of opinion between scientists as to the precise nature of the muck in the protein. A very vocal majority is convinced that it is precisely and uniquely the HIV virus. A smaller group thinks that generalized abuse of the body opens the way to any number of opportunistic infections, including HIV.[7]

Pam Francis of *Today* was curious and enthusiastic about the programme's subject, and Sheridan Morley wrote intelligently in *The Times*, 'There can no longer be anything so simple as the "HIV equals AIDS equals death" belief. It [AIDS] has become a commercial as well as medical issue and its complexities have only begun to be fully appreciated by a medical press which has, until recently, been too willing to accept official government reports.'[8] Christopher Dunkley in the *Financial Times* said our programme took the orthodoxy 'by the neck, shakes it vigorously, and sets off to see what the calm thinkers outside the multimillion dollar research lobby are saying. The result is eye opening.'[9]

Then the big guns waded in. A letter published in the *Independent* from the All Party Parliamentary Group on AIDS, signed by Lord Kilmarnock and 18 others called the programme 'irresponsible' and 'a source of grave concern for anyone involved in health education and the prevention of the spread of HIV'. 'The programme appeared to be a quite deliberate attempt to discredit the efforts made by those who attempt to educate the public about risks of HIV infection and should not in our opinion have been transmitted as it stood.'[10]

Channel 4 continued to be supportive. David Lloyd captured the essence of the position in reply to the *Independent*:

For as long as the HIV *hypothesis has held sway, a small but not insignificant minority of medical science has dissented. These people are not cranks, still less are they discredited. Indeed, in the two years since Dispatches first reported on* AIDS, *their number has grown. A lay public has not been told this. In the thousands of hours of broadcasting reporting upon, or predicated upon, the* HIV *hypothesis, there has been not a mention. Against this,* Dispatches *has placed two 40-minute broadcasts. A lack of balance? When those programmes that identify themselves with mainstream opinion are prepared to grant the minority a voice, then* Dispatches *will be guilty of imbalance in not seeking out replies from the majority.*

Professor Walter Gilbert of Harvard concluded the programme with these words: 'The great lesson of history is that knowledge develops through the conflict of viewpoints. If you have simply a consensus, it stifles.'[11]

Our most bitter disputes were both with and in the letters pages of the *Independent*, the *Independent on Sunday* and the *Guardian*. Steve Connor, a science journalist, was in the middle of writing a book about AIDS. He was totally immersed in the virus/AIDS hypothesis. Any questioning of that hypothesis could pose questions about the validity of his book. Over the next two years he would be unrelenting in his animosity, taking every opportunity to try to discredit Duesberg and our efforts to open up debate. Connor decided to highlight complaints from two distinguished scientists, Max Perutz and Sir Aaron Klug, both Nobel laureates working at the MRC's Cambridge laboratory of molecular biology. They were also deeply involved in a number of MRC HIV research projects through the Cambridge laboratory at the time. Klug questioned whether television was the right forum for debate on such a complex technical subject,[12] while Perutz took his attack to the *Guardian*: 'Many of those who watched it [the programme] may now throw precautions to the wind and contract the most sinister, terrible disease to afflict mankind since the plague.'[13]

Duesberg shot back a reply: 'Regrettably, the panic about HIV generated by numerous unbalanced AIDS-virus programmes that have "failed to give a platform to scientists and doctors who could have expressed these facts ..." has infected even the scientific elite at Cambridge.'[14] Perutz returned another volley:

I cannot understand the insensitivity and thoughtlessness of the people who produced this programme and who allowed it to be transmitted. Have they ever seen an AIDS patient? ... If I were a producer and thought by assuring people that AIDS is not infectious there might even be a very small risk of my being wrong and of some people who believed me contracting AIDS, I would tell myself that by showing such a programme I would commit a terrible crime and I would desist. They did not.[15]

Duesberg spat back:

As was pointed out in the programme we all agree with Perutz that safe sex is a valid protection against contagious venereal diseases, like syphilis and gonorrhoea. However, there is currently no evidence that such measures will prevent AIDS, and there is no evidence that a sexually transmitted infectious agent is capable of causing AIDS. Even if there is just a chance that AIDS is not infectious, this should be seriously discussed both publicly and among the health scientists, because many lives are at stake and not one has been saved by the expensive virus/AIDS hypothesis.[16]

Here again is the moral ambiguity of an orthodoxy that does not allow a conflicting hypothesis to be discussed openly. Morality, it seems, can be enlisted to support an orthodoxy, but where was the morality in perpetuating a hypothesis that might simply be wrong? That the prevailing infectious hypothesis could in itself be preventing the truth from emerging, thus blocking new avenues of research that could help resolve the puzzle of AIDS, did not seem to have a morality value.

Duel with *Nature* and Koch's Postulates

The fiercest duel since transmission of *The AIDS Catch* was between

Duesberg and John Maddox (now Sir John) then editor of *Nature*.
Maddox has always refused to publish a paper from Duesberg. Yet he
has peppered his journal with deeply critical and often offensive pieces
about Duesberg's position on AIDS. Sir John Maddox was as stubborn
as Duesberg was tenacious. I saw him as a Toby jug figure, with Duesberg, the German schnautzer, snapping at his ankles and Maddox, all
English phlegm, beating him off with his stick.

After *The AIDS Catch*, Maddox published an article called 'Duesberg,
HIV and AIDS' by Robin Weiss and Harold Jaffe. Both Weiss and Jaffe
claimed to have isolated their own strains of HIV. The tone of the
article was derisory from the start. They called Duesberg 'absurd' and
criticized *The AIDS Catch* for not attempting 'to state the evidence for
the mainstream, scientific view that it sought to demolish'.[17] Their
attack focused on the fact that Duesberg maintained that the virus/AIDS
hypothesis did not fulfil Koch's postulates, a series of principles
devised by scientist Robert Koch to identify whether diseases are
infectious or not.

Koch was one of the founding fathers of microbiology, and it was he
who first identified the cause of tuberculosis. His postulates lie at the
heart of Duesberg's arguments and need to be explained. Robert Koch
was an eminent German scientist who, in the last century, laid down
the criteria that would enable us to identify an infectious agent.

Duesberg had long maintained that molecular biology and hence
retrovirology has spiralled downwards into a chasm of reductionism.
The more scientists saw under the microscope the more mistakes they
made as they tried to attach what they were seeing to specific diseases,
often blaming them as infectious agents. Koch was important, said
Duesberg, because he laid down criteria for infectivity that needed to
be met. These criteria are not met for HIV. The four postulates are:

- *The germ (infectious agent) must be found in the affected tissues in all
  cases of the disease and in amounts sufficient to cause pathological
  effect.* No HIV at all can be isolated from 10 to 20 per cent of AIDS
  patients. HIV cannot be isolated from the cells in Kaposis's sarcoma
  lesions, nor from the nerve cells of patients with AIDS dementia.

And too few HIV infected cells are ever found in the body to cause damage.

- *The germ must be distinguished from other germs and isolated from the host's body.* There is so little HIV in AIDS patients that the only way the virus can be identified is indirectly, by taking huge amounts of cells from that patient and then reactivating the virus. In classical diseases enough active virus is present to be isolable directly from the blood or affected tissue. One million to 1000 million units of virus per millilitre of blood can be found during the time most viruses cause disease – for example in active hepatitis infection or pneumonia. Not so with HIV. It is usually found in less than five units and never in more than a few thousand units per millilitre of blood plasma. Duesberg states that such low quantities are insufficient to cause disease. It is only when the amount of virus in the body is high enough to overwhelm more cells than the body can regenerate rapidly, that a disease condition occurs.

- *The germ must cause the sickness when injected into healthy hosts.* HIV has never caused disease when injected experimentally into chimpanzees, nor when accidentally injected into human health care workers.

- *The same germ must, once again, be isolated from the newly diseased host.* Until the third postulate, that the germ (HIV) causes disease in a new host is confirmed, this postulate cannot be tested.

The importance of these criteria in differentiating between an infectious and a toxic agent came clear to me when Duesberg compared the London cholera epidemic in the mid-nineteenth century with the Spanish olive oil poisonings. Both were examples of clusters of people dying from an unknown pathogenic agent. The first turned out to be infectious, the second toxic.

It was Dr John Snow, a Hampstead physician who with Sherlock Holmes-like skill found out what was affecting his patient living near Hampstead Heath. Snow has been hailed as the first epidemiologist –

epidemiology being the study of the pattern and spread of disease. Snow's patient was the only Hampstead resident who had developed the terrible cholera symptoms. She liked the waters from the Seven Dials pump in Covent Garden so used to send her horse and cart down there every day. Snow knew that people who lived around the Seven Dials pump were dying like flies from fever, vomiting and diarrhoea. Why was she the only patient with these symptoms in Hampstead? He followed her horse and cart down to the pump and tore the handle off – no more cholera epidemic.

In Spain, when the olive oil tragedy broke out, hundreds of people became paralysed and died. Others suffered lifelong nerve damage. The agent was believed to be illegal contaminants in batches of olive oil, probably combined with the effects of certain pesticides used in the region.

These two examples show two clusters of disease. By applying Koch's postulates you would have been able to tell immediately that the Seven Dials pump disease was caused by an infectious agent. The germ, a living organism, could reproduce itself in the body and infect others as well. It would have been found in all victims. It could be isolated, and it could cause the same disease if injected into healthy hosts. The case of the Spanish olive oil was an example of intoxication, or poisoning. The active toxic chemical agent could not reproduce itself. It was not therefore infectious.

If we replace the cholera germ with HIV in the first story we will find that HIV cannot be the infectious agent that causes AIDS because it can meet none of the postulates. However, if we compare the clusters of victims from the Spanish olive oil disaster, with the clusters of AIDS cases in New York, San Francisco and other large cities where drug taking and promiscuous gay sex abound, then the high risk/toxic hypothesis for AIDS becomes utterly tenable.

In their *Nature* article, Weiss and Jaffe acknowledged that Duesberg was right on two of the four postulates, but said that he was wrong on the first. Their argument on the first postulate was that although Duesberg maintained that HIV was found to be active in only 1 in 400 T-cells – too few to cause any damage – HIV *may* (my emphasis) be found in other cells like bone marrow and lymph nodes and that Duesberg is ignoring indirect mechanisms for T-cell depletion. Weiss and Jaffe then said that the postulates were now outdated and did not apply to viruses. The problem was that Weiss and Jaffe were talking about hypothetical reservoirs of infected cells and 'indirect mechanisms' that were not known and therefore unproven. Duesberg worked from what was known and proven. Weiss and Jaffe continued, 'In the face of compelling epidemiological data causally linking HIV with AIDS, one need not harp upon molecular quibbles. ... To deny the role of HIV in AIDS is deceptive.'[18] Such blind faith in epidemiological data is risible. To quote Duesberg again, 'Association [the fact that HIV is *there*] does not prove causation.' The article went on to call Duesberg 'perilous', 'belittling of safe sex' and 'a flat earther bogged down in molecular minutiae and miasmic theories of disease.'[19]

Duesberg wrote a careful 1700-word rebuttal entitled, 'Weiss, Jaffe and the germ theory of AIDS', and submitted it to Maddox. 'I submit the enclosed rebuttal expecting equal space and terms as "Commentary" to *Nature*. It was written in the same Popperian spirit of hard hitting, scientific sportsmanship as the Weiss-Jaffe challenge, to illuminate and defend statements made by myself, but also those made by Meditel, Gilbert and others in *The AIDS Catch* programme.'[20] Maddox flatly refused to publish it.

Duesberg wrote to complain enclosing a revised version of his paper saying, 'I have been called "absurd", "amply refuted", "perilous", "confusing". ... I find it very insensitive of you to tell me that I am "ungenerous" toward the authors of the article. ... Have you considered that this article is damaging to my professional reputation and thus libellous if not at least balanced by an equivalent refutation?'[21] Still Maddox wouldn't budge. He finally restricted Duesberg to a meagre 300-word letter. In it Duesberg wrote:

As a virologist, I understand their [Weiss and Jaffe's] fascination with infectious agents. However, it is romantic, not scientific to abandon proven rules like Koch's postulates without providing new ones to accommodate HIV as the cause of AIDS. Thousands of lives have been lost in the past because medical scientists, inspired by successes of the germ theory, have misdiagnosed as infectious diseases vitamin deficiencies, like pellagra in the US, or scurvy in England and recently a drug induced neuropathy in Japan.[22]

There were other colleagues who lobbied Maddox on behalf of Duesberg at this time. Beverly Griffin, Director and Professor of virology at the Royal Postgraduate Medical School, Hammersmith Hospital, wrote to Maddox to complain about the way Duesberg had been treated, but with no reaction. She later wrote a paper to the *Lancet* which was rejected. In it she said:

In steadfastly maintaining his position, Duesberg and his standing as a scientist have been undermined, and in Nature *he was pilloried in an article to which he was allowed only limited reply. That scarcely seems 'cricket' but this is not the issue. If he is totally wrong, he may deserve some of the criticism that has been heaped upon him, but the point is, we don't really know if* HIV *causes* AIDS, *nor have we really seriously tried to find out.*[23]

Joseph Schwartz, a physicist trained at Berkeley and author of the book *Creative Moment*,[24] also wrote to Maddox saying:

After ten more years of research, we may know everything there is to know about HIV *and still be left with* AIDS. ... *I hope* Nature *will give Duesberg the space to present what experiments/studies he thinks could decisively settle the issue. The stakes are much too high to tolerate the present public relations exercises with name calling and ridicule taking the place of a serious exchange of views.*[25]

His letter was never published. The deadlock between Maddox and Duesberg continues to this day and has had some curious twists and turns. Suddenly, in September 1991, Maddox wrote an astonishing editorial called 'AIDS research turned upside down'. He wrote, 'Professor Peter Duesberg from the University of California, Berkeley is probably sleeping more easily at night now than for five years, since he first took up cudgels against the doctrine that AIDS is caused by the retrovirus HIV.'[26] Two important pieces of research had prompted these remarks. The most important was a study from Vancouver that showed that animals, never exposed to any HIV risks, when injected with HIV free blood tested antibody positive for HIV. The significance of this will become clear in the last chapter of this book when we discuss the hypothesis that HIV itself is not an entity in itself but is simply identified through a series of proteins said to be specific to HIV.

When Professor Geoffrey Hoffman in Vancouver discovered that his laboratory mice, never exposed to HIV or any other agents, developed HIV antibodies when injected with foreign HIV-free lymphocytes, he was perplexed. How could this be? This study would turn out to be of key importance in explaining why HIV itself was, at this stage in the history of AIDS, being wrongly identified as a retrovirus.[27]

We had been alerted about Hoffman's work and I had spoken to him over the telephone. He said he could not really explain his findings, but, interestingly, he said he would like to be able to do a further study. He speculated that women who had had several children by the same man, if exposed to foreign sperm, would react in the same way as the mice, developing 'antibodies' to HIV yet remaining perfectly healthy.

The second experiment Maddox referred to was conducted by E. J. Stott in the UK. It showed that monkeys that had not been vaccinated against SIV (simian immunodeficiency virus, which is believed to be analogous to HIV) had developed their own defence against attempts to infect them with the virus. The explanation offered by the research team was 'that AIDS is an essentially autoimmune disease in which T-cells have lost the normal "anti-self" interdiction but instead kill each other'.[28]

Maddox wrote: 'Duesberg has been pilloried for his heterodox views . . . and faced with the threat that his research funds would be snatched away. Now there is some evidence to support his long fight against the establishment (among which, sadly, he counts this journal.'[29] This was indeed a welcome turn of events. Was there at last a tiny crack in the AIDS edifice? Alas, no, a more recent episode reveals that Maddox, angered by Duesberg's contention that AIDS is related to intravenous and long-term recreational drug use, decided to commission an article that would once and for all put paid to this heresy. He asked Professor M. S. Ascher to write it.[30] (A separate article along the same lines by M. T. Schechter in Vancouver appeared that same week in the *Lancet*.)[31]

The Ascher article claimed that in a study of mostly homosexual men from San Francisco, the incidence of AIDS diseases over eight years was independent of drugs and that 'when controlled for HIV serostatus, there is no overall effect of drug use on AIDS'.[32]

Duesberg tore into the study saying it was 'worthless'. He criticized Ascher and his colleagues for not taking the consumption of AZT into account, but his strongest criticism was of the graph in the study. It contained six curves. One of the curves was said to represent HIV positive people who did not take drugs. Duesberg's scrutiny of the study showed that there were no HIV positives in the study who did not either inhale poppers (nitrites) or use illicit drugs like cocaine and amphetamines. This curve, he said, represents nobody and is therefore a fabrication.[33]

Outrage! One scientist was accusing another of a fabrication. Maddox absolutely refused to publish Duesberg's response and wrote a very curious piece, this time headed 'Has Duesberg a right of reply?' 'What is to be thought of a science journal that publishes attacks on the opinions of a scientist but which never (or hardly ever) publishes his replies?' he said. 'On the face of things this is a serious breach of journalistic ethics. ... How can such intolerance be justified?' Maddox accused Duesberg of 'making demands' and of asking 'unanswerable rhetorical questions'. He continued:

Duesberg has forfeited the right to expect answers by his rhetorical technique. ... The truth is that a person's 'right of reply' may conflict with a journal's obligation to its readers to provide them with authentic information. ... Duesberg will not be alone in protesting that this is merely a recipe for suppressing challenges to received wisdom. So it can be but Nature will not use it. ... When he offers a text for publication that can be authenticated, it will if possible be published – not least in the hope and expectation that his next offering will be an admission of recent error.[34]

It might, perhaps, be possible to understand Maddox's position a little better if he had received an unsolicited article from Ascher, but the fact that he actually commissioned it in advance makes his subsequent stance appear very unfair indeed.[35] It is almost comical to note that he refers readers to the rival the *Lancet*, where Duesberg had finally managed to get a reply published.

So the *Lancet* did publish a reply and the accusation that Ascher had fabricated an 'empty set' of figures to represent 'seropositive-no drug use' did stay in. Duesberg added, 'To refute my hypothesis Schechter [who had written the *Lancet* article] and Ascher would have to produce a controlled study showing that over a period of up to ten years HIV-positive individuals who use recreational drugs or zidovudine or both have the same AIDS risks as positives who do not do so.'[36]

The Edinburgh AIDS Conference – Pilloried in Public

Whenever any of our team was invited to speak in public about our programmes, we set out with well-rehearsed scientific arguments and high hopes that we might get a good hearing. We were always disappointed. But we never expected the public humiliations that invariably took place, engineered by the very chairmen and women of the groups who had invited us. Edinburgh was one of the worst.

In August 1990, the forty-fourth Edinburgh International Film Festival decided to organize a one-day 'AIDS and the Media Event'. We were invited to participate at the last minute as it became clear to the director, David Robinson, that our film *The AIDS Catch* was to be the focus of debate. He hadn't been able to find anyone to support our film so why didn't Michael Verney-Elliott and I, the makers of the film come up? I invited Jad Adams to join us and we set off. We thought at the very least our film would be shown. It was a film festival after all.

We soon discovered that our participation was far from welcome. The panel included Duncan Campbell, the broadcaster Sheena McDonald and panel chairman, Derek Ogg, also chairman of Scottish AIDS Monitor. We were never called to speak but were fiercely criticized. After a series of ill-informed contributions from the panel, Duncan Campbell took the stage. He produced no scientific arguments to support his case against us. He called us 'murderous' and me a 'cheat' for having duped Professor Luc Montagnier and epidemiologist Dr Andrew Moss into appearing in our film (both willing interviewees, who had been made fully aware of the approach of our programme.)

Jad Adams began a prepared speech but was interrupted. Adams protested that he had been invited and should be allowed to finish. Derek Ogg said words could not describe the way he felt about our presence. He said he had not invited us, neither would he ever have had us on the panel. So much for impartial chairmanship.

We should have learned our lesson, but accepted another invitation to speak at a Bristol conference organized by the Avon Health Authority. This time it was the women who turned on me. Several young women who had been drug users had tested positive. Their status had made them queens in their locality. They were famous and they were receiving a great deal of financial support from the local health authority. They should have wanted to hear the good news – that HIV did not necessarily carry a death sentence with it. But no, completely conditioned – or better, brainwashed – they preferred the death sentences that supposedly hung over them than to question the assumptions that underpinned their 'treatment'. Forming a menacing circle around me they spat out their taunts and venom.

Defunding the Dissident: Duesberg Sidelined

More bad news followed. Duesberg had been the recipient of one of the most prestigious research grants in the USA – an outstanding investigator's grant from the NIH – worth $350,000 a year over seven years. The time came for him to apply for a renewal. His application for further research into retroviral oncogenes, cellular proto-oncogenes and some separate research on AIDS was turned down. He was told he had spent too much time on the AIDS debate and had not published enough original papers. A panel of his peers, although referring to Duesberg as 'one of the pioneers of modern retrovirology', judged that he had become 'sidetracked' and could 'no longer be considered at the forefront of his field. . . . More recent years have been less productive, perhaps reflecting a dilution of his efforts with non-scientific issues.'[37]

Duesberg was incensed. He wrote back to say that he had published countless papers and letters and papers on the AIDS debate which were highly original. He was particularly concerned at the choice of the reviewers for his grant application, and had discovered through a chance telephone call that, of the three reviewers he himself had put forward because he deemed them 'unprejudiced', although listed as reviewers, two of them had not presented a review at all and the third had delivered a review by phone which was much more favourable than the score listed in the letter of rejection from the NIH. In a letter to Dr John Cole at the NIH Duesberg wrote:

> *By selecting reviewers who hold views and have commercial interests that are in direct conflict with my application, those at the NIH who selected the panel for my application could make or break it. ... Therefore the selection of Dani Bolognesi and Flossie Wong-Staal – whose well known professional careers are mainly built on AIDS research – for the review of my application, would generate a very predictable method of '[impacting] the priority score given to [my] grant application'.*[38]

It was all to no avail. He was defunded. Over the next two years, Duesberg lost his secretary and his postdoctoral students. His faculty bosses at Berkeley decided he should no longer teach graduates, so he was allocated an undergraduate laboratory course. He was, in fact, academically emasculated.

The Broadcasting Complaints Commission: Interest Groups on the Attack

Lady Anglesey sat across the narrow table from us with her handsome face and perfectly coiffed hair – one of the 'great and the good'. On her left and right were other august members of the Broadcasting Complaints Commission (BCC) – a panel including a lawyer and an ex-broadcaster. They were there to pass judgement on us; not to discuss the finer points of science, mind you, but simply to judge whether or not we had been 'unfair' in our treatment of AIDS. How could we possibly be judged fairly, we protested, if we were not allowed to put forward the scientific arguments in our own defence? These formed the very basis and justification of our programme. Besides, science had nothing to do with fairness. It was about fact.

It was all a sham from beginning to end, and today the grounds upon which some of the complaints were entertained by the BCC are no longer allowed. However, this was no laughing matter. The whole process took over a year and many months of work for us, reading and drafting documents together with Channel 4's tireless lawyer, Don

Christopher. The way the establishment manipulated the BCC was entirely transparent. There were two complaints hearings. The first, held on 14 March 1991, was on behalf of Wellcome, the makers of AZT. The second, 12 days later, involved a joint complaint from three AIDS organizations, the Terrence Higgins Trust, Frontliners and Positively Women. The Terrence Higgins Trust had received funds from the Wellcome Foundation, produced four booklets about AIDS including one about AZT together with Wellcome and, as a charitable AIDS organization, promoted the use of AZT. The trust seemed almost duty bound to come in fighting its patron's fight. The Wellcome Foundation accused us of being one-sided, of making damaging remarks about their product AZT, of expressing an unorthodox view, and of not accurately presenting the current consensus of medical opinion.

On our side of the table at the hearing were David Lloyd and Don Christopher from Channel 4, journalist John Lauritsen (who had flown over from New York for the hearing) Michael Verney-Elliott and myself. Wellcome argued from the basis that its drug AZT had been approved after scientific trials. We knew we had documents, obtained through the US Freedom of Information procedure, that showed that these trials (funded entirely by Wellcome) had been prematurely terminated, were deeply flawed and that at one trial centre at least data had been tampered with by their own representative. But this was not what the BCC was interested to hear. The panel wanted none of the facts and none of the scientific background.

Wellcome's representatives put up a poor show. There was one good moment when Lady Anglesey rebuked Wellcome for not being able to provide any follow-up mortality data on the men who had taken part in the trials that led to the licensing of AZT.

We fought our corner hard and came out feeling very optimistic. But the Commission eventually judged that we had 'unfairly treated the subject of AIDS', and of being 'unfair to Wellcome' on three out of four counts. David Lloyd said later 'It was like winning a football match ten nil and then being told later that you had lost!' The BCC said it did not consider that it was unfair for the programme to give expression to an unorthodox view. However, they agreed with our accusers on the following three points:

- *That there was unfairness in the programme's failure to indicate the relative strength of the medical and scientific opinion against Professor Duesberg's thesis.* (We had pointed out from the start of the programme that we would be making a challenge to current accepted orthodoxy.)
- *That we misled the viewers in our criticism of* AZT, *by saying that no one had lived longer than three years on* AZT, *without making it clear that* AZT *had only been generally available to the public for three years.* (The BCC missed the point here that our criticisms stemmed back to the use of AZT in patients who had participated in the trials long before AZT came on the market.)
- *That we should have used the interview with Professor Ian Weller and included comments of his like 'I don't think the level of toxicity is unacceptable.'[39]* (Our reasons for not including the Weller interview are explained earlier.)

The next hearing, held on 26 March 1991, involved the three AIDS organizations. Duncan Campbell had been asked by the Terrence Higgins Trust's director, Nick Partridge to represent the Trust.* We were kept waiting an hour while a video Campbell had prepared was shown to the panel. This had never been done before, so the BCC did not know what to do, but finally agreed to view it on the very morning of the hearing. Campbell had interviewed some of the people in our film and provided a highly edited stream of complaints. But with Montagnier, who never did complain, Campbell had cleverly used a clip from our film and added his own commentary saying that

---

* In January 1992 the Charities Commission launched a formal inquiry into the financial dealings of the Terrence Higgins Trust. There had been four chief executives in four years. The charges of fraud and corruption revolved around Nick Partridge, acting chief executive, on a salary of £31,500 a year. Partridge had announced at an extraordinary staff meeting held at the Trust's Gray's Inn Road headquarters on 28 October 1991 that 11 staff would have to be laid off 'owing to financial difficulties'. The organization's financial policies were then questioned, in particular the payment of £115,000 to an outside fundraiser, Andrew McDonald. After 17 months little or nothing had been raised. It also emerged that £78,000 of staff pension monies had been used to meet staff salary costs. Former chief executive, John Fitzpatrick said that the Trust 'has become a gravy train for AIDS careerists' (*News*, No. 3, January 1992).

Montagnier had been unfairly treated and misrepresented. The overall impression given was that Montagnier himself had complained. When I brought this to the attention of Lady Angelsey later, she ticked Campbell off.

We were all ushered into the conference room and shown the video, and the session was opened. The Terrence Higgins Trust accused us of 'directly undermining and diminishing the effectiveness of efforts by ourselves and others to limit the spread of HIV infection and to relieve suffering'. It also accused us of causing harm and suffering because 'false claims' in the programme had led people to refuse to take AZT. They said the programme makers were 'reckless as to the likelihood that unnecessary deaths were a probable consequence of their programme', of knowingly including statements that were wrong and of unfairly editing our interviewees.[40]

The upshot of this highly unsatisfactory charade of a hearing, dominated by Nick Partridge and Duncan Campbell, was that a month later we were found guilty on three out of four counts regarding interviewees: of misrepresenting the views of Montagnier, Moss and Friedman Kien, but not those of 'Anna' from Positively Women. The adjudication concluded that, '*The AIDS Catch* was likely to have misled many viewers about the present consensus of medical and scientific opinion on AIDS and confused them about the risk of HIV infection through unprotected sex.' The BCC found that this was 'unfair'.[41]

There were moments of nobility in all of this. Channel 4's support for us was unwavering. Don Christopher, Channel 4's lawyer, said the BCC's verdict was 'one of the most disgraceful judgements the BCC has ever made'. And the Independent Television Commission (previously the IBA) said the programme had been clearly labelled as one side of the argument, and that 'the discretion involved in editing the interviews of contributors had been exercised fairly'. They declared that: 'If the views put forward in *The AIDS Catch* had been wrong, the appropriate response was to refute them with better arguments and better evidence. To suppress them, as the Terrence Higgins Trust seemed to want, would have been unscientific and illiberal.'[42]

Chapter 8

'AZT: Cause for Concern'

AZT: AIDS by Prescription

The fundamental truth about the research establishment is that the scientific community feels that it shouldn't have to answer to the rest of us. So the notion that a non-scientific person would go on and question the research that they used, the accuracy of their data and the truth of their interpretation, provoked a tremendous controversy throughout the research establishment.

(Elinor Burkett, journalist)[1]

H e walked slowly into the HEAL office, a dissident AIDS support group, in Manhattan's lower east side. He had a black patch over one eye, a gold embroidered cap on his head. His black skin glowed against the peacock green of his flowing African robes, hiding his painfully thin body. Alan Roundtree had AIDS. This was 1991 and we were in the middle of filming our third programme on AIDS for Channel 4's *Dispatches, AZT: Cause for Concern*. Alan had been prescribed AZT, the only allegedly anti-AIDS drug on the market at the time. He felt so ill he had had to stop taking it. In all ten years of interviews on AIDS this young man's words, more than anyone else's, have remained ingrained in my memory:

At first I gained weight and I said, 'Boy this stuff must be working'. And then about another two weeks later it did start working. The headaches came. The dizziness, the nauseousness. I had fingernails so black it looked like I had nail polish on. The upset stomach. Nothing tasted right. You couldn't listen to people because you didn't want to hear them because you were hurting so bad. It left me impotent. It destroyed my hopes for living.[2]

AZT was the only existing drug indicated for AIDS. It was also being given to HIV positive people with no symptoms of AIDS. Yet, in spite of the manufacturers claiming that it prolonged life and delayed the onset of AIDS, doctors actually working with patients could only see them getting sicker and sicker before their very eyes and then dying.

Why? Quite simply, AZT is a DNA chain terminator. That means it destroys the mechanism by which new cells are made in the body. It stops the growth of DNA causing the fast or slow death of the immune system because all growing cells will be killed by the incorporation of AZT. Its action is similar to cancer chemotherapy, whereby bad cells are killed in the hope of keeping enough good cells to survive. In cancer chemotherapy the treatment is given for a limited period of time. AZT is prescribed indefinitely – until death.

Other evidence supporting irreversible damage from AZT had been published in the *Lancet* in 1988. Drs Christine Costello and Naheed Mir reported serious bone marrow damage in their patients on AZT, with 36 per cent requiring blood transfusions. The authors write, 'It is worrying that bone marrow changes in patients on zidovudine (AZT) seem not to be readily reversed when the drug is withdrawn. . . . These findings have serious implications for the use of zidovudine in HIV positive but symptom-free individuals.'[3]

Apart from inhibiting DNA synthesis and killing healthy cells, AZT (according to Wellcome's own official literature) has other serious effects on the body. It causes severe disturbance of the gut, accompanied at times by projectile vomiting. It produces unendurable headaches, muscular atrophy, destroys bone marrow and causes severe anaemia, often requiring blood transfusions. Hundreds of thousands of young men with the AIDS syndrome were swallowing up to 1500 milligrams a day of these blue and white capsules, and continuing to feel desperately ill.

AZT was first developed as a cancer chemotherapy drug in 1964 (to kill unwanted cells). However, it was considered too toxic as a cancer drug and discarded. Some 20 years later, Wellcome applied for a change of use for AZT as an antiretroviral drug. The claim was that AZT could target HIV infected cells and home in on them when reverse transcriptase activity takes place. That is when, according to the orthodoxy, the enzyme called reverse transcriptase, which a retrovirus like HIV needs in order to knit itself into its host cell, goes into action. This action, called reverse transcription, converts the retrovirus's RNA into its host cell's DNA – its genetic blueprint.

Two trials using patients, called phase I and phase II (described later), were conducted before AZT was licensed for the treatment of AIDS. Journalists in the USA were way ahead of the UK on the subject of AZT's toxicity and the doubts surrounding its use. As far back as 1988 John Lauritsen had begun to write his series of articles critical of AZT[4] as had Celia Farber.[5] Dr Joe Sonnabend had publicly stated that AZT was 'incompatible with life'. Michael Ellner and Frank Buianouckas of HEAL, New York, had registered strong protest about the drug's toxicity and of course Duesberg had by now alerted the scientific world of his grave concerns in his second *PNAS* paper[6] and in 'The role of drugs in the origin of AIDS'.[7]

In 1988, Perri Peltz made a series of reports critical of AZT on NBC News. All of this went on in the USA. Precious little had been said in the UK, even though Wellcome, which made the drug, was a British company. Two important early pieces, critical of the drug and of the way the AZT trials had been conducted, appeared by Brian Deer in the *Sunday Times*.[8] Duncan Campbell also went into print about the pricing and marketing of AZT in a *New Statesman* article entitled 'The AIDS scam'[9] where he criticized Wellcome's monitoring of AZT side effects such as muscle disease.

As soon as we received the green light from David Lloyd at Channel 4 to begin work on AZT: *Cause for Concern*, we plunged into the debate. This was October 1991. In our research phase Lauritsen had sent us two sets of documents from the US Food and Drug Administration (FDA) obtained through the US freedom of information procedure. One set had been requested by an AIDS pressure group in San Francisco called Project Inform and the other by John Lauritsen himself. They were powerful evidence indeed of the gross irregularities that had gone on during the Wellcome-funded trials that led to the licensing of AZT.

After an initial very small trial called phase I, the phase II AZT trials were set in motion. A total of 282 AIDS patients were recruited, roughly half being put on AZT and the other half receiving the placebo (dummy tablet). These were the trials that led eventually to the licensing of AZT as an AIDS drug. They took place in 12 study centres across the USA and it is on the basis of their findings that all future justification for the use of AZT rests. The studies were grossly flawed. Irregularities were found at all trial centres and in one that the FDA investigated, in Boston, 'The FDA inspector found multiple deviations from standard protocol procedure and she recommended that data from this centre be excluded from the analysis of the multicentre trial.'[10] However, these concerns were cast aside at a series of FDA meetings where it was agreed to include all data, bad and good, 'Because the mortality analyses were so strongly in favour of the drug, any slight biases that may have been introduced when minor "protocol violations" occurred were highly unlikely to influence the outcome.'[11]

It was the mortality figures reported in the phase II trials that led to the trial's premature termination in 1986. The figures purported to show that while there were 19 deaths in the placebo (non-AZT) group there was only one death in the drug group. We shall analyse these figures later. After the Boston trial centre, under the supervision of Dr Robert Schooley and Wellcome's monitor Ron Beitman, was investigated, the FDA investigator, Barbara Spitzig's 76-page report reveals an astonishing list of breaches of protocol.[12] The study was not properly blinded; that is, by sending their tablets to be tested at independent laboratories, the patients knew who was on the drug and who was on the placebo. Chris Babick of the People with AIDS coalition had confirmed this to us when he explained how his organization had referred people in the phase II trials to three laboratories in New York to get their tablets analysed. If they discovered they were on the placebo they would arrange to buy AZT. If they were on AZT they would share their drugs with those on the placebo.[13] Other breaches in protocol involved the altering of patients' original forms. They had been altered and symptoms crossed out or otherwise changed, usually without the principal investigator's initials. The FDA report includes phrases like, 'the sponsor [Wellcome's Beitman] unfairly biases against the placebo group', and 'the sponsor makes the analysis look more favourable to AZT.' The report says, 'Adverse experiences were sometimes crossed out months after initially recorded, even though "possibly related to test agent [AZT]" had been checked off by the investigator or his designee'.[14]

The trial supervisors failed to report adverse reactions in many patients on AZT. For example, patient 1055 suffered fatigue, nausea, loss of appetite and was admitted to hospital with a fever of 105°F. His form said he had experienced no adverse reactions. It was not possible to check the way pill bottles were labelled because Beitman had picked up all the empty and full bottles the week before the investigators arrived and he had destroyed them all. The study supervisors received money according to the length of time a patient was in the study. The Boston centre report contained lies about the length of time many of its participants had remained in the study.

The real bombshell was the story surrounding patient 1009. When Lauritsen received the set of FDA documents he had requested through the freedom of information procedure they had black splotches all over them, where they had been censored. However, the censor failed to cover up the fact that patient 1009 had been on AZT *before* entering the trial, was very ill, and had to be given blood transfusions, but he was entered into the placebo group. When he later died, his death was counted among the 19 placebo deaths.

Harking back to the mortality figures (19 in the placebo and one in the drug group) that led to the early termination of the trial and the eventual licensing of AZT, patient 1009's case shows that already the figures needed to be changed to 18/placebo 2/drug. And this was an investigation into only one of 12 trial centres. The abiding faith I had had, until then, in the type of trials that were considered to be the gold standard in science – double-blind placebo-controlled trials* – ended the day I read Lauritsen's evidence.

---

* These involve studying two groups, one taking the real drug and the other taking a dummy tablet or placebo. In order to 'blind' the trial, neither the patients nor their doctors know who is taking the drug and who the placebo. This should allow a clear assessment of the drugs benefits and risks.

AZT Phase II Trials: Mortality Figures Manipulated

It is the allegedly indisputable evidence of AZT's effectiveness as reflected in the mortality figures that is always quoted as the reason why AZT 'works'. But 30 of the group on AZT had been so badly affected by the drug that they needed blood transfusions to keep them alive by the time the study was terminated. These 30 would have died from anaemia anyway because they did not have enough red cells of their own left and needed to be transfused with red cells from other donors in order to stay alive. In the placebo group there were five cases of anaemia. These could have been due to AZT because the trial had become unblinded, trial participants had had their tablets independently analysed and patients on AZT were misguidedly sharing their tablets with those who had discovered they were on placebo, thereby rendering the trial invalid.

Duesberg worked out that if you included the 'would be' deaths in the AZT group (in other words those individuals who suffered such severe effects from AZT that they would have died had they not been kept alive with blood transfusions), a far higher number of deaths would have featured in the group that was given AZT. Instead of one, it would have been 31 (1 plus the 30 who had needed transfusions). In the placebo group, the numbers would also have been different. Instead of 19 it would have been 24 (the original 19 plus the 5 who presumably developed AZT-induced anaemia from the drug sharing). He compared these figures statistically. Instead of only one death in the AZT group and 19 in the placebo group, the figures were now 31 and 24. 'Now', he said, 'there is no longer room for celebration.'[15] It is important to know that within weeks of the trial being stopped a further 10 per cent of the patients who had been on AZT, died. Lauritsen writes:

I regret not having previously characterized the AZT trials as fraudulent. I do so now. Fraudulent is by no means too strong a word to use in describing a study which was prematurely terminated for specious reasons, in which false data were deliberately retained, in which cheating was tolerated, and in which improprieties and violations of protocol were delib-

erately ignored. It is fraudulent to describe an unblinded study, which the
AZT *trials most certainly were, as being a 'double blind' study, as principal*
investigators Margaret Fischl and Douglas Richman did in their reports in
the New England Journal of Medicine. *Either Fischl and Richman were*
unaware that the study had become hopelessly unblinded, in which case
they are guilty of incompetence, or they did know and covered it up, in
which case they are guilty of fraud.

If someone set out to make wine, and instead ended up with vinegar,
what should he call the final product? Wine or vinegar? Obviously vine-
gar, because that's what it is. Nevertheless, Fischl and Richman, and their
confederates in the FDA, the NIH and Burroughs-Wellcome, persist in
calling the unblinded AZT *trials a 'double-blind, placebo-controlled' study.*[16]

AZT and Cancer

Among the documents the FDA were asked to release under the
Freedom of Information Act was a review carried out by Dr Harvey
Chernov, submitted on 29 December 1986.[17] Chernov reviewed
numerous studies including in vitro experiments with rats, mice,
rabbits, beagle dogs and humans. He noted that AZT was toxic to bone
marrow, causing anaemia, and that AZT was found to be weakly
mutagenic in the mouse lymphoma cell system. In addition, chromosomal damage was observed. Evidence from the 'cell transformation
assay' (invariably carried out using human cells), indicated that AZT
was likely to cause cancer. In his summary, Chernov wrote, 'This
behaviour is characteristic of tumour cells and suggests that AZT may
be a potential carcinogen.'

Chernov was genuinely concerned that in the rush to approve AZT,
the FDA was proceeding on the basis of inadequate information. 'FDA
guidelines would have prescribed more extensive preclinical testing
than that reported thus far. However, the urgency for developing an
anti-aids drug has been so great that the clinical testing has preceded
the usual/customary pre-clinical testing.' Chernov recommended that
AZT should not be approved for marketing: 'In conclusion, the full
preclinical toxicological profile is far from complete with 6-month
data available but not yet submitted, one-year studies to begin shortly

etc. *The available data are insufficient to support FDA approval* [emphasis added].[18]

In his *New York Native* article 'AZT and Cancer' John Lauritsen writes, 'Samuel Broder of the National Cancer Institute (NCI) is the man who is more responsible than anyone else for the development and promotion of AZT. Even Broder now admits that his drug may cause cancer. He is coauthor of a recently published article in the *New England Journal of Medicine* (*NEJM*) in which it is stated: 'In considering early intervention with zidovudine (AZT) it is of particular concern that the drug may be carcinogenic or mutagenic; its long-term effects are unknown.'[19]

A further concern about AZT arose when it was noted that patients on it for up to three years were developing an increased incidence of non-Hodgkin's lymphoma, a virulent cancer of the B-cells produced in the body's lymph nodes. A study by Dr Robert Yarchoan showed that up to three years on AZT suggested a 46.4 per cent estimated probability of developing lymphomas.[20] Although Yarchoan et al. state that profound immune suppression can lead to lymphomas, they conclude, however, that 'a direct role of the therapy itself cannot be totally discounted. As improved therapies for the treatment of HIV infection and its complications result in prolonged survival, non-Hodgkin's lymphoma may become an increasingly significant problem.'[21] This was the state of affairs when our team set out to discover what patients and doctors on the front line of AIDS were thinking about all of these problems.

AZT: Cause for Concern: Structuring the Story

Arriving for the flight at Heathrow and seeing all those gleaming silver boxes full of camera, sound and lighting equipment is always a joy. All those weeks of research, budget adjustments and itinerary planning over, I could actually see the technical 'means of production' before my own eyes. Ian Owles, our camerman, and Chris Renty in charge of sound, were bent double checking their flight case labels and taping locks and corners against bumps and scrapes. At last the whole team was together.

I had decided to construct the film around the four major claims about AZT made by Wellcome in its own literature, which we knew to be false. By quoting claims made by Wellcome itself, we would be on strong legal ground. A promotional booklet issued by Wellcome to doctors and the general public states:

- 'There are no life-threatening toxicities associated with zidovudine [AZT]'
- 'none of the volunteers or clinicians involved [in the various AZT trials] knew who had received placebo and who had received the active drug'
- 'zidovudine improves both quality and length of life'
- The booklet also states that AZT is an antiviral drug and gives the impression that AZT can target the HIV virus without damaging uninfected cells.[22]

The film would challenge all these statements and find them to be false. This meant that if successfully prosecuted Wellcome would be guilty of a criminal offence, namely that of making false claims about its drug.

In San Francisco, Duesberg gave us of his best. He not only claimed that AZT does not work because it cannot be selective and kill HIV without killing the whole of the HIV-infected cell and other good ones with it, but also that HIV has never been shown in humans to present a meaningful target for AZT. To understand these assertions we need to remind ourselves how the current orthodoxy describes the way a retrovirus like HIV works.

Current orthodoxy maintains that retroviruses like HIV are made of RNA (ribonucleic acid). When they enter a new cell they need the DNA of their host cell in order to survive. They can be described as cell dependent scavengers. To knit themselves into their host cell's DNA they have to go through a chemical process making use of an enzyme called reverse transcriptase. HIV can then knit its RNA into the DNA – the genetic heart – of the cell it is invading, quietly take up residence there and lie dormant without destroying its host. It becomes a harmless passenger. Wellcome claims that AZT can target HIV when the process of reverse transcription is taking place – in other words, before HIV has knitted itself into its host cell's DNA. But Duesberg points out, as we shall see, that because HIV is dormant most of the time, there is hardly any further infection with HIV taking place, which means there is hardly any reverse transcriptase activity going on. So there is no target for AZT.

Why AZT Does Not Work

The fundamental life-giving process of cell regeneration depends on DNA, which is made up of four building blocks that slot together. One of these is called thymidine. AZT is a copy or analogue of thymidine which, when it attaches itself to the viral DNA chain, stops it because nothing else can attach itself thereafter. It is as if a train wagon has lost its coupling (the next wagon cannot attach itself so slips away) – thus Duesberg's description of AZT as a DNA chain terminator.

Wellcome claims that AZT can target HIV and delay symptoms of AIDS in people who are HIV positive by inhibiting HIV when reverse transcriptase activity takes place (immediately after the virus gets into the cell). Duesberg maintains that AZT cannot be selective and cannot prevent the virus from infecting that cell without killing it and non-infected cells as well:

In people who are given AZT, healthy or sick, only one in five hundred cells is ever infected by HIV. That is to say in order to kill one infected cell, we have to kill five hundred normal cells, good cells that people, particularly with AIDS desperately need to survive, and healthy people need them too. It is like trying to kill a terrorist in a city like Berkeley of 200,000 by poisoning the water. You may get the terrorist, but you will get most of the other people as well.[23]

But does AZT have a viral target at all? Duesberg maintains that once a person has developed antibodies to HIV, the virus becomes inactive. It is lying dormant in its host cell, not moving out to infect other cells, and not triggering the reverse transcriptase activity it would require to do so. So, essentially, there is no target for AZT because there is no reverse transcription going on. 'There's no evidence for it. It's not detectable, and the number of infected cells remain the same, it remains very low, and remains constant, which is direct proof that further infection is not taking place. Further infection depends on reverse transcription.'[24]

San Francisco General Hospital is perhaps the most famous AIDS hospital in the world and is the home base for one of the leading proponents of AZT, Dr Paul Volberding. He, together with Margaret Fischl at Miami University (whom we were to visit later in the shoot) co-wrote the controversial phase II trials and was also involved in subsequent trials that led to the licensing of AZT in people with no symptoms of AIDS.[25]

A tall good-looking man with a boyish face, Volberding ushered us into his office at the top of the AIDS unit building. He displayed consummate skill in sliding out of the more difficult questions and clung to his view that AZT therapy should be started early 'before the patient becomes so advanced that the side effects become intolerable'. On whether he thought the use of AZT could be justified he said, 'I think the question increasingly in the United States is not whether to use it, but whether to use it by itself or whether to add other drugs to AZT.' (This was hardly a good advertisement for the effectiveness of AZT, we thought.) His further justification of the phase II trials on the issue of unblinding was no more reassuring: 'I don't think it's completely true that the trial was unblinded. In retrospect there are ways that we could have known who was taking the drug. The drug causes the red blood cells to enlarge in size. But that wasn't really known at the time and so I think that the trial was in fact quite well blinded.'[26]

This half-hearted support for the validity of the phase II trials certainly did not impress us as we headed for San Diego to meet Professor Charles Thomas. Charles Thomas was well known to us. He had founded the Group for the Scientific Reappraisal of the HIV/AIDS hypothesis, which had grown into a membership of 200 (later to grow further to 500) scientists and health professionals who question the virus/AIDS hypothesis. The group's journal *Reappraising AIDS* was beginning to be read by and to influence more than just the converted. Thomas, an ex-professor of biology at Harvard, had moved to San

Diego to run his own company of laboratory diagnostics and was now in the thick of the AIDS debate.

I considered myself to be one of the .01 per cent of Americans that [sic] could read and understand the scientific papers that were purported to document that HIV is the cause of AIDS. . . . And what I found there was not a very convincing argument. . . . Our group is trying to achieve one thing. We want the critical experiment that will prove or disprove the HIV hypothesis done – not just talked about after ten years. We want to compare HIV positive and HIV negative individuals in terms of their prospective mortality and morbidity. For example, to this day we don't know whether HIV causes people to become sick or not. Just think of it.[27]

On AZT he said:

I think there are two things wrong. First of all it's highly doubtful in my mind that HIV causes AIDS. And secondly, even if it did, it would be a lousy way to kill that virus. First of all the virus is only infecting such a small fraction, perhaps 1 in 500 of the lymphocytes. Secondly, only a small fraction of them, 1 in 10,000 are actually producing a message or are active in any way, and when you apply AZT, this is a chain terminator and is directed against the totality of the replicating genome. So the target size is enormous. There's a million kilobases of DNA in a human cell and there's only ten kilobases of HIV, so that represents only one part in 10,000 and it's a ridiculous way to approach chemotherapy of a virus infection.[28]

When we caught up with Robert Hoffman, Professor of Cancer Biology at the University of California in San Diego, he put a further disturbing spin on AZT. Hoffman told us that apart from preventing cells from replicating, those cells that survive AZT may themselves become cancerous.

I believe that the drug AZT can have at least two important areas of toxicity and that is the inhibition of production of critical white cells and also the production of malignant cells such as lymphoma cells. These two

121

courses can be monitored but they can also reach the point of no return where nothing can be done about it. So even with monitoring, these toxicities can be life-threatening.[29]

So much for Wellcome's claim that there are no life-threatening toxicities associated with AZT.

The US Veterans' Administration Study on AZT

Raleigh–Durham, North Carolina is an important place. These adjacent towns house one of the biggest pharmaceutical research complexes in the world as well as the renowned Duke University founded with money from the tobacco magnates. Raleigh is also the headquarters of Burroughs Wellcome, its massive building looking like a white blancmange sprawled across a vast expanse of landscaped and manicured lawns. We knew we would be unable to interview anyone at Burroughs Wellcome. Our requests for interviews in the UK and USA had been rejected. In the UK Martin Sherwood, Wellcome's group public relations manager, had written to us saying:

In view of your public refusal to accept criticism of your programme-making by a respected and independent body, the Broadcasting Complaints Commission, we regret that we are unable to believe that you are sufficiently balanced and objective in your approach to the subject of AZT to make a reasonable programme about it. Consequent to this view, neither we nor our colleagues in Burroughs Wellcome, USA, are prepared to participate in your programme.[30]

Tucked away in a corner of Duke University campus in a bungalow-style building one of our key interviewees awaited us. It was with Dr John Hamilton, who had conducted the longest ever trial of AZT (three years) on people with AIDS and early symptoms of AIDS. His paper was published the day after the transmission of our programme.[31]

The Hamilton study was funded by the US Veterans' Administration (VA) and was based at Duke University. The VA is an impressive organization that looks after the needs of all veterans of the US armed forces. Any medical research entered into by the VA has a vast pool of people to draw from and is rigorously executed.

Hamilton was a 'gentle' man in every sense of the word, yet he was sitting on a volcano. The study design was to give AZT to an 'early' (less ill) group and to a 'late' group with T-cell counts below 200. The results of his study showed that there was no difference in length of survival between the early and late groups and that there were more deaths and more multiple AIDS diagnoses in the 'early' group that took AZT longest. This was the group, remember, that was less ill at the beginning. Being less ill they would have been expected to live longer than the more ill. Instead, they died at the same time. Their deaths had been accelerated. To put it at its simplest, the group that was less ill but took AZT longest, got sicker and died quicker.

The study did say that 'early zidovudine therapy slowed the progression to AIDS', but these men still did not live longer than those who had been given AZT much later on in their illness. How could this be? There seemed to be a contradiction here. On closer questioning off camera, Hamilton revealed that he had had to say that because the results of the phase II trials (the trials that had led to the licensing of AZT) had shown such dramatic benefit in the mortality figures (challenged earlier in this chapter) and he felt he had to give due recognition to these findings. But, looking at me meaningfully he said that he had no idea what the 'delayed progression' benefit meant in terms of time. 'It could be a day,' he said, with as close to a wink as he dared.

On film, Hamilton told us that the blood disorders caused by AZT are potentially life-threatening and went on to say, 'I think it is self-evident that our study does not provide the kind of benefit that everyone wished for. It can't be a secret that patients wanted something that would help them live longer. ... Unfortunately it has not demonstrated that and therefore this has to be unwelcome news.'[32] So much for Wellcome's claim that AZT prolongs life. On quality of life, Hamilton said:

There has been no formal demonstration in quality of life. It was assumed that the delay in progression to AIDS would translate into an improved quality of life because it seemed logical and made sense. In fact the only

123

study that has been done on this point and published to my knowledge has
failed to demonstrate an improvement in quality of life.[33]

Hamilton was referring to the work of Dr A. Wu. His first study into
quality of life in people with AIDS showed no difference in terms of
mobility and physical and social activity between those on AZT and
those on a placebo. Wu's second study, on people with 'early symptomatic HIV infection' showed that the patients on AZT had an inferior
quality of life compared with those on a placebo in terms of overall
health, well-being, energy, mental health and pain.[34] So much for
Wellcome's claim that AZT improves quality of life.

If ever there was evidence that AZT did not prolong life, did not
improve quality of life and caused more harm than good here it was.
But how to convince the world of this? It was Miami and Dr Margaret
Fischl's turn next.

The Queen of AZT Trials

Dr Margaret Fischl was a leading light in the two key trials
surrounding AZT: phase II, which led to the licensing of the drug for
AIDS, and the NIAID (National Institute of Allergy and Infectious
Diseases) trial, which led to the prescribing of AZT to people with no
symptoms of AIDS. She has been described as 'the wicked witch of AZT'
but she greeted us with a smile, attempting to radiate certainty.
Fischl's attempt to explain her position was muddled and confused.
Here was a scientist in the grips of a tussle between her own scientific
integrity and her loyalty to her paymasters, Wellcome. 'Once it enters
the cell,' Fischl explained, 'the drug [AZT] has to undergo a transformation so it becomes active and then it actually *prevents* [emphasis
added] the virus from infecting that cell. ... It prevents the cells from
becoming infected but it does nothing for cells that are already
infected.'[35]

But what of the view that AZT cannot possibly prevent a cell from
becoming infected without killing the whole cell? Fischl stated
repeatedly and categorically that AZT did not harm non-infected cells.
This directly contradicted Wellcome's own published literature in

drug information journals for doctors on AZT's side effects, which stated that AZT killed bone marrow cells, and others.[36]

Not surprisingly, Fischl went on to deny that her phase II trial had become unblinded and claimed that AZT prolonged life and improved quality of life, making 'the patient's life more productive'. But she did add that in future combined drug therapy might be better with other drugs similar to AZT like ddI (dideoxyinosine) and ddC (dideoxycytidine). And if others came along that attacked 'the AIDS virus differently from AZT, then those combinations would be superior'.[37] Once again, this was not a very good advertisement for the wonderful efficacy of AZT.

New York: AIDS Dissidents Speak Out

We met Dr Michael Lange at St Luke's-Roosevelt Hospital in New York. His kind face and unlimited energy in caring for patients with AIDS had established his reputation as a dedicated physician. He had also become angry. None of his patients had got better on AZT. He had been one of the AIDS doctors who had cooperated, in good faith, in the trial Margaret Fischl and others had conducted that led to AZT being given to people with no symptoms of AIDS.[38] However, he was unhappy about the way things turned out and believed the trial was terminated too early to be of any use.

He reminded us that this trial was supposed to last three years but was terminated when the patients had only taken the drug for a mean period of nine months. Said Lange: 'Now to me it stands to perfectly good reason that if you stop a study with placebo, using a drug where you knew previously that there may only be benefits for six months, if you stop that after nine months, you will definitely bias the study towards AZT.'[39] The licensing of AZT in 1990 for HIV positive people with no symptoms of AIDS, he believed, was a gross error. He was also incensed at the way AZT was being advertised by Wellcome in poster campaigns. The posters encouraged people to get tested for HIV and said, 'Early medical intervention could put time on your side.'

As AZT was the only approved drug for AIDS at the time, this was a way of increasing Wellcome's market for the drug. 'I think it's a disgrace,' said Lange. 'It lures people into the belief that if they're HIV positive they should go and get themselves tested and there's an answer that will keep them alive, and that's far from the truth.'[40] Another poster showed three small children racing across a lawn. The poster read, 'Helping keep HIV disease at bay in children'. Retrovir (the brand name for AZT) is written in big letters and, above it, 'Generally well tolerated. Improved cognitive function. Survival rates similar to adults. Improvement in growth and well-being.'

Lange also had strong views about the emergence of lymphomas in patients taking AZT. He disagreed with Volberding's view that lymphomas were a late manifestation of immune-suppression and a natural consequence of living longer with AIDS (and therefore not AZT related). 'Almost all the lymphoma that I have seen,' said Lange, 'was a first AIDS event and occurred not at the late stages of the disease but was the diagnosis that was made that made that patient an AIDS patient. And prior to AZT coming along I never saw lymphoma in people who had had several opportunistic infections as a late stage event.'[41] What pained Lange most was that he saw his patients rally for a while on AZT with rising T-cell counts which then plummeted.

I would say that in most cases, or in a number of cases you do see a small increase in T-4 cells during the first three to four months. Usually by six to nine months, if you're lucky by twelve months, you're back to where you started from. And from there on there's in most cases a general decline so that you end up with T-cells less than beforehand.[42]

But what could be causing this apparently beneficial rise in T-cell counts early on in therapy, which then seemed to cancel itself out? Dr Harvey Bialy helped us out. As science editor of *Bio/Technology*, the sister paper to *Nature*, Bialy had had a great deal of experience of the 'science' surrounding AIDS. He was one of the few editors who had resisted publishing articles that unquestioningly accepted the virus/AIDS hypothesis.

A brilliant molecular biologist and friend and colleague of Duesberg's, he had spent many hours batting the HIV/AIDS arguments backwards and forwards over the telephone with him. On the temporary rise in T4 cells, he told us:

I don't know that one needs to explain it more than by noting that the rise is very temporary. This is not uncommon when a body is shocked by a toxic assault of one kind or another – for the metabolic system to go into a high gear for a while and compensate for the initial insult. But the fact that these rises in T-4 cells have never been seen to persist – that a drug produces an initial clinical response and then that response disappears to be replaced by clinically damaging responses does not speak well to the therapeutic index of that drug.[43]

With the weight of scientific evidence that had built up surrounding the danger and inefficacy of AZT, why were its critics not listened to? In the words of Celia Farber, a New York journalist who had worked extensively on the HIV and AZT story:

In the beginning there was a near religious devotion to it [AZT]. It was very emotional. There was this idea that anybody who criticized AZT was doing it for all the wrong reasons. Either for publicity or for some kind of hidden agenda. I think with some of the leaders of the gay community, what happened was they were on AZT and while it was working for them they were much more stridently arguing for it. Then, as you know, it has a grace period, then it drops off and it really doesn't work any more and then it backfires. And when they got to that stage in their AZT therapy they just had to turn round and say, 'Hey, you know this stuff doesn't work. It's no good.' And that's really where it's at right now. ... There's almost nothing to hold on to any more. I really don't hear anything other than – well, yes it's a terrible drug but it's all we have.[44]

London: AZT and the Gay Community

Cass Mann had founded his AIDS support group Positively Healthy in 1987. Many of the group's members were young gay men who had been diagnosed HIV antibody positive. Some had early symptoms of AIDS and others were asymptomatic. Disillusioned with AZT, they had decided to look for alternative ways of keeping healthy, without receiving orthodox anti-AIDS medication. Under Cass Mann's leadership, Positively Healthy had been very active over the past year and had published detailed information for its members on the background to the AZT story and on the dangers of its toxicity. What happened when his members came off AZT, we asked Cass?

When they come off AZT you obviously have some people who go through a period of withdrawal. There are the various side effects that take time to wash out. But generally, I have found in my experience that people after a month or six weeks coming off AZT regain their health. It's not just coming off AZT. We put them on various co-therapies like nutritional therapy, vitamin and mineral therapy, traditional Chinese medicine etc., to support the immune system. And I can say in almost every single case we have a recovery which is quite remarkable. ... Over 95 people have come off AZT since 1987. Many of them have come off it for a period of three years. They're all doing extremely well. They've regained their health. They're living a full and normal life.[45]

This group of HIV positive men who were surviving well without AZT would have provided a valuable research cohort (group) for anyone genuinely interested in comparing their progress with patients on AZT, but sadly the research purse strings have been so dominated by Wellcome and the MRC that no money has been available for any genuinely alternative avenues of research. It has taken over a decade for the group to persuade its area health authority to conduct a study called the Park Project, looking into the possibility that HIV may not cause AIDS and instead examining nutrition and lifestyle factors in both HIV positive and negative men who are considered to be at risk.

When, in 1989, after the trials in asymptomatic patients were terminated early and it was announced that AZT could be used not only for people with AIDS diseases but for a much larger group – with HIV and low immune cell counts but no other symptoms, Wellcome's shares soared to new heights adding £1400 million to the company's UK stock market value in one day. By 1991, when we were making our programme, the annual sales of AZT were worth £170 million worldwide. By 1996 annual sales of AZT had reached £200 million.

It was at this time that Professor Ian Weller gave a progress report on his findings of the Concorde trial, the Anglo-French study looking

at the effects of AZT on some 3000 asymptomatic HIV positive participants. Weller gave his report on Concorde at a meeting held at the
Terrence Higgins Trust. Cass Mann, representing Positively Healthy,
one of the voluntary groups at the meeting, recorded the proceedings
and we used excerpts from this recording in our programme. Weller
argued the case for continuing the trial but at the same time he made
some astonishing admissions:

*It seems to me that the Data and Safety Monitoring Committee feel very
comfortable in allowing this study to proceed into what I think is new
territory – and my feeling is that it's that territory that most patients and
physicians are interested in. That is if there is benefit is it maintained or
will it wear off? In which case we may be doing more harm than good
[emphasis added].*[46]

Professor Weller then said the monitoring committee found no clear
evidence on which to base new recommendations for clinical practice
and that the trial into AZT would continue for a further seven months.

*My feeling is that this is the only chance that anyone will have for sorting
out the uncertainty that I think is at the basis of some of the frustration,
that is whether it is better in the mid to long term rather than short term,
to give zidovudine (AZT) early or rather leave it to a later stage of
infection? Early intervention does make biological sense. The question,
the pragmatic question, the practical question is, do we have the right
tool [emphasis added]?*[47]

It seems incredible that with all the evidence already available to him
on AZT's toxicity and ineffectiveness, Weller wanted to continue
involving 3000 people for another seven months in a study when he
did not know if he was doing 'more harm than good' or whether he
was using the 'right tool' at all.

Magic Johnson Shrugs off AIDS

There was further research to be done before the final rough cut of the programme could be made. It was during the final stages of our programme editing that the Magic Johnson story broke. Here was one of America's greatest heroes, king of basketball, and self-confessed womanizer with thousands of sexual partners during his career, stricken with HIV. Everyone wanted to make use of Johnson's predicament to further their own ends. Here was the perfect vehicle to get the safe sex message through to heterosexuals, thought the health educators. Here was the perfect man to encourage everyone to get tested and get more people on to AZT, thought Wellcome and the AIDS doctors. 'Experts hope the announcement by Magic Johnson will encourage people who suspect HIV infection to get tested because treatment is most effective in early stages' cried *USA Today*'s front page.[48]

Johnson had just closed a deal with the Lakers' team making him one of basketball league's highest paid players ($2.5 million for the 1991/2 season). Johnson was quoted to this effect in the *Observer*:

The doctors then said that because the physical and emotional rigours of the 82-game Laker season might weaken my immune system, just as the virus would, they were recommending that I retire from professional basketball. I honestly didn't give it a second thought. ... The following day I stood at a podium at the Great Western Forum, the place where I had some of my greatest moments as a Laker – and spoke from my heart. I said that because I had tested HIV positive, I was retiring from the NBA [National Basketball Association].[49]

As far as his health was concerned he said his physical condition never changed and that he felt completely healthy. 'I was actually in the best shape of my National Basketball Association career and, at 32, was about to start my thirteenth season with the Lakers.'[50] That was in October 1991. But almost immediately he started on AZT things changed dramatically. A report two months later in the US press said he had lost his appetite and was suffering bouts of nausea and fatigue. 'I don't have the energy I once did,' said Magic, 'and I feel like vomiting almost every day. When I think about this, I just want to grab Cookie and take her in my arms and blot out the world.'[51] The symptoms Magic was suffering were the classic symptoms of AZT toxicity.

However, the orthodoxy, through pure conjecture, attempted to manipulate Magic's situation to make him fit the mould. It was reported that Magic may have had HIV for years, which was why his T-cells were at 500 and that he was likely to begin suffering full-blown AIDS sooner than he expected and that he should have been put on AZT months ago. In the same article, Dr Howard Temin is quoted as saying that when an infected person's T-cell level drops below 500 'it means the virus is getting better and the immune system is getting worse.'[52] Since hardly any trace of virus is ever found, commented Duesberg, how can the virus be 'getting better'?

Then rumours began to emerge that Magic had stopped taking AZT. Whatever the truth, he certainly stopped having the serious side effects he had described in late 1991. Then, in the first months of 1992, Magic made a remarkable recovery. He began to play again, closely monitored by his doctors. 'And when nothing changed,' he said, 'when I was still able to run and do everything without getting tired, then that settled that. It put my mind at ease.'[53]

He was selected to play in the 'dream team' for the Barcelona Olympics and began to tour with the Magic Johnson All Stars raising money for his AIDS foundation. On 30 January 1996, the world press reported that Magic Johnson had rejoined the NBA and was playing with his old Lakers' team that very day against the Golden State Warriors. A report said that some NBA players had refused to play with him in the past because of his HIV positive status and that he was turned down for an exhibition match in the Philippines for fear their players would become infected. But all of that had changed. I watched the match on television. Magic looked bigger and fitter than ever and the Lakers' team won.

After the initial high doses of AZT that made Magic feel so ill his treatment was changed and he was put on a cocktail of drugs including *some* AZT, a reverse transcriptase inhibitor and a new drug called a protease inhibitor (see Chapter 14). His doctors have since announced that the virus in his bloodstream is below detectable levels.[54] So far, Magic's constitution is able to tolerate his AZT-reduced drug regime well.

We held a press viewing of the programme and were finally ready for transmission. But on the day before transmission Liz Forgan, Channel 4's Director of Programmes, received a letter from Professor Ian Weller:

I am led to believe that a 'secret' tape recording of myself addressing representatives of the voluntary organizations at the Terrence Higgins Trust is used in the programme. ... I am led to believe that the programme makes serious allegations and reaches potentially damaging conclusions. ... I would ask you to assure me that my contribution to this programme will be removed. I would also urge you consider the harm that this programme might do to those patients infected with HIV and to those currently on treatment.[55]

Having declined to participate in our programme, Weller was perhaps understandably anxious that he should not be misrepresented through selected quotes at his Terrence Higgins Trust meeting, but his letter went further with its suggestion that the programme might cause harm, and is demonstrative of the pressure the medical establishment can bring to bear on television executives in order to prevent transmission of any challenge to the medical consensus. As in all cases when disputes arise surrounding controversial programmes, this one was referred up to Channel 4's then head of factual programmes, John Willis. He said it was a 'strong story' and approved the programme for transmission. It was transmitted on 12 February 1992.

Wellcome's Claims about AZT

The last statement in our film said, '*Dispatches* has been advised by leading counsel that the false and misleading claims about AZT described in this programme could amount to a breach of the Medicines Act, which, if successfully prosecuted, would constitute a criminal offence. *Dispatches* is sending a dossier of relevant information to the Medicines Control Agency at the Department of Health.'

In the final stages of our production, Channel 4's lawyer Jan Tomalin consulted a QC regarding our programme's evidence alleging that Wellcome was making false and misleading claims about AZT. Under section 93 of the Medicines Act it is a criminal offence to advertise or promote a product in a way 'likely to mislead as to the nature or quality of medicinal products ... or as to their uses or effects.' A legal precedent had been set in 1986 when the pharmaceutical company, Roussel, was prosecuted by the Department of Health for making false and misleading statements about their non-steroidal anti-inflammatory drug Surgam. Roussel were found guilty and appealed, but were eventually convicted. They had to pay a fine and prosecution's appeal costs.

The QC told us that we had a very strong case and that she believed it would hold up in court. We therefore sent our dossiers off to Dr Susan Wood at the Medicines Control Agency (MCA) and to Professor William Asscher at the Committee on Safety of Medicines. At first Dr Wood at the MCA expressed anger that we had not handed our information over to them before transmission of the programme. Certainly, no editor could do such a thing for fear of transmission being blocked through attempts at injunctions.

Three weeks later we received a brief dismissive letter from Dr Wood saying that AZT had undergone 'rigorous assessment and consideration by the licensing authority and its expert advisory committees prior to licensing. Other regulatory authorities throughout the world have reached similar conclusions on the benefits and risks of the drug.'[56] The fact that it was precisely these decisions that we were questioning had obviously passed Dr Wood by.

We had no luck from the Committee on Safety of Medicines either. Professor Asscher wrote back to say that advertising was nothing to do with them. 'Our role is to advise on the licensing of medicines and thereafter to monitor adverse drug reactions.'[57] Again, the fact that our programme and the dossier we sent him were all about licensing and adverse reaction issues had obviously passed him by too. We then learned that the MCA and the Committee on Safety of Medicines had had their government funding reduced and were now partially dependent on fees from the pharmaceutical industry for their survival. So much for vigorous independent watchdogs.

There was an explosive reaction to our programme after transmission. Accusations surfaced from every direction, not least over the telephone. We had grown used to this. A whole year after our criticism of AZT in *The AIDS Catch*, Phyllida Brown had called from the *New Scientist* to ask me how I felt about the fact that our programme had made many patients stop taking AZT. 'How do you feel about that?' she demanded menacingly, implying that I was of course causing their deaths. Her call had followed a survey conducted by Professor Brian Gazzard at St Stephen's Clinic in London revealing that some of his patients had suspended their AZT treatment after that programme. Gazzard said patients' reactions to the programme demonstrated 'the need for great caution in deciding whether or not a TV programme [of this kind] should be made'.[58] Then had come the very unpleasant call from Duncan Campbell who hurled both professional and personal insults at me. He was quite unable to discuss any points of science and could not bring himself to admit that there might be something wrong here, especially after the results of Dr Hamilton's VA study. His harangue centred on my gross irresponsibility and my being a danger to his friends with AIDS.

I again wondered how scientific inquiry could ever make progress on the AIDS issue when it was so heavily embellished with emotion. The emotive response of commentators laced with the self-interest of so many scientists and researchers made for a literally deadly mix.

Defending AZT: Wellcome's Damage Control

Our programme was transmitted on the same day as publication of Hamilton's VA study in the *New England Journal of Medicine*.[59] John Lauritsen was the first to fax us over the news agency reports about Wellcome's shares. They had dropped 17 pence ahead of transmission. Needless to say, after the programme went out, Wellcome, with its huge financial resources behind it, went into a brilliant public relations exercise in damage control.

With the transmission date of our programme in mind and only nine days before it went out, Wellcome had already issued a 'Dear Doctor' letter to every GP in the land, announcing the results of an AZT trial called EACG 020, which it had financed itself, in low risk asymptomatic HIV infected people. The trial was chaired by Professor D. A. Cooper in Australia and once again this trial had been suddenly terminated. It claimed that 'disease progression was significantly reduced' and that 'the serious side effects seen with zidovudine when used in advanced disease appear to have been virtually absent in this study.'[60] This was a perfect example of science by press release. The study had not been peer reviewed or published and was shortly to be discredited by AIDS specialists in the scientific journals. But how could a hard working, well-meaning GP have known the background to all of this?

When the EACG 020 study was eventually published in August 1993, Brian Deer wrote in the *Sunday Times*:

[AIDS specialists] have accused Wellcome researchers of misleading the scientific community following the publication of a report that appeared to show AZT was effective in AIDS prevention. Leading doctors expressed outrage at what some regarded as a public relations stunt by Wellcome. The company's study [EACG 020], they said, was old, flawed in its methodology and had been terminated before anything meaningful could be reported.[61]

Even our old adversary Phyllida Brown wrote in the *New Scientist* of Wellcome's 'mischief-making and of being disingenuous in its portrayal of the findings.'[62] To keep up the pressure after transmission of our programme, Wellcome issued a second 'Dear Doctor' letter. It landed on GPs' desks saying, 'You may have seen the *Dispatches* programme which was transmitted on Wednesday 12 February 1992. ... We are writing to you now because we believe that it may cause unwarranted distress to some of your patients.'[63] The letter then offered information that 'will help you to provide a balanced assessment of the current situation for your patients with regards to HIV infection and its treatment with zidovudine.'

Then came the letter from Wellcome's chief executive, John Robb to Channel 4's chief executive, Michael Grade. Robb immediately launched into an attack about the BCC and a personal attack on me, 'When the Commission upheld our complaints, Ms Shenton of the production company Meditel publicly denounced the BCC, despite having participated fully in its complaints procedure.' Robb went on to describe his company's high standards in the quality of its medicines and in its claims for them, which 'in no way build false hopes'. He continued, 'We find it deplorable that your company [Channel 4] does not seem willing to apply similarly high standards of quality control when entering the public arena on these highly emotive issues.'[64]

Michael Grade's response was swift. On Robb's comments about the BCC he said, 'I should remind you that it was not only Ms Shenton of Meditel who criticized the finding. To this day the Independent Television Commission continues to stand by the programme and its methods and Channel 4 itself has declared that on this issue the BCC had 'strayed beyond its normal area of competence into one in which it was extremely difficult for it to be seen to adjudicate fairly.' It is to be regretted that the Wellcome Foundation declined Ms Shenton's invitation to participate in the more recent programme; in the 13 years of her company's existence, Meditel has won seven major television awards including the Royal Television Society's Journalism Award.' Grade ended his letter saying:

You write of the need to maintain standards and to avoid building false hopes – on these highly emotive issues. I cannot but agree with you. It is in this spirit that our own legal department were advised by leading counsel that they should advance the programme's research to the Medicine's Control Agency and the Department of Health – so that they should be able to judge for themselves whether the claims made on behalf of AZT could be judged false or misleading – at law.[65]

Wellcome's next move was to write a letter to the *Lancet*. Dr D. S. Freestone of Wellcome Research Laboratories started his letter off with – yes – the mention of a 'previous programme by the same television production' company that had 'shown little sensitivity to the needs of patients and prescribers, and it had been found by the independent Broadcasting Complaints Commission to be misleading, confusing, unbalanced and unfair and to misrepresent the views of some experts.'[66]

But I was grateful to Dr Freestone because it gave me the opportunity to reply in the *Lancet*. I was able to justify our stand against the BCC and to home in on the mortality data from the phase II trials with an important piece of extra information:

These trials planned for 24 weeks were terminated after an average of only 17 weeks. In the 21 weeks after the trial ended and the drug became available to all participants, 10 per cent of the patients on zidovudine died. Furthermore, when zidovudine became available on a compassionate plea basis survival statistics were kept on 4805 patients. David Barry of Burroughs Wellcome commented to journalist John Lauritsen (24 May 1988) that somewhere between 8 per cent and 12 per cent of AIDS patients treated with zidovudine died during four months (17 weeks) of treatment. If in a similar period of 17 weeks less than 1 per cent died during the phase II trials yet 8–12 per cent died following release of the drug, then the most likely explanation is that the [trial] figure is unreliable.[67]

Some nice things did happen. We had two very fair reviews, one by Tony Delamothe in the *British Medical Journal* and a piece in the *Lancet's* Noticeboard, which I suspect was written by Dr Richard Horton. And we won an award! None other than the BMA awarded our programme a certificate of educational merit.

However, we were not even able to enjoy this little fillip for long because we were soon to hear that the Terrence Higgins Trust had launched into an attack on the BMA for giving us the award, saying it should not have endorsed a programme that presented a minority view and neglected the strong scientific evidence offered by the other side.[68] Complaints about our position on AZT from AIDS charities like the Terrence Higgins Trust were no accident. 'As sales of AZT have grown – last year reaching £213 million – the company has extended its own funding and support operations to a huge range of AIDS organizations, including a parliamentary group [the All Party Parliamentary Group on AIDS] to which it has contributed £65,000,' wrote Neville Hodgkinson in the *Sunday Times*. 'Critics say the result has been to foster a climate in which the antiviral approach to AIDS has squeezed out almost all other lines of inquiry.'[69]

Defending a Dissident: A Scientist's Fair Play

Channel 4's *Right to Reply* gives viewers a platform to air their criticisms about a programme. I was invited to take part by a researcher. I asked who would be against me and I was told 'a concerned GP'. What *Right to Reply* failed to tell me was that the 'concerned GP', Dr Simon Mansfield, was a senior doctor at the Kobler centre, a specialist AIDS clinic attached to the then St Stephen's Hospital. We later discovered that Dr Mansfield was actually taking AZT at the time. He died a few months later. Before he died, Mansfield had written to Dr John Hamilton enclosing a copy of our programme already converted to the American NTSC standard. (We had of course already sent Hamilton a courtesy cassette of the programme.)

His letter began by referring to the publication of Hamilton's VA study in the *New England Journal of Medicine*. It went on:

You may know that Joan Shenton is a controversial figure in British broadcasting, especially since following her last programme made on the subject of AIDS and HIV she was admonished by the Broadcasting Complaints Commission for misrepresenting the people that she had interviewed.

The programme that she recently made for Dispatches *was controversial. Your involvement in it was very interesting indeed and I wonder if you could spare the time to review this video of the programme which I have converted into the American system. I would be most interested to know if you feel that your views have been fairly represented in the film. I am not sure that the conclusions which the documentary comes to are in line with your important paper ... I am considering making a complaint to the Broadcasting Complaints Commission about her programme and I would be most interested in your reaction to it.*[70]

This was blatant sycophantic trawling for more people to complain about us to the BCC. Hamilton's response to Mansfield was uncompromising:

I was unable to review the video you sent me as it was damaged and would not play. I had received, however, a copy of the Dispatches *program from Miss Shenton somewhat earlier.*

They did ask difficult, controversial questions – questions that merit debate in most cases. Overall, those of my views that were telecast were not selectively chosen it seems to me. Inclusion of the data derived from our VA study for discussion was entirely appropriate. ... I think it is unfortunate that Burroughs Wellcome, both USA and UK, were unwilling to be interviewed as I believe their perspective is very important. ... In summary I am satisfied with my own contribution to the program as it was televized and feel that the treatment of the general issues was somewhat more adversarial than desired but not unacceptably so.[71]

Chapter 9

Amsterdam and All That

The Amsterdam Alternative AIDS Conference: Dissidents Gathering

It was a glorious week in May and Amsterdam was having a heat wave. A group of us were staying in a small hotel near the Rode Hoed, an old wooden church bordering one of the canals in the heart of Amsterdam, which was the conference venue. The church, once a refuge for religious liberals, was opening its doors this week to the largest gathering ever of AIDS dissidents, their critics and the press. One of the most important aspects of the conference, entitled 'AIDS – A Different View', was that it had been able to attract leading members of the AIDS orthodoxy. Our old adversary, John Maddox, editor of *Nature* would be there, and Luc Montagnier was expected the following day. The Dutch AIDS establishment was well represented by scientists Jaap Goudsmit, Roel Coutinho and Frank Miedema.

The evening we arrived the dissident factions gathered together in our hotel cellar bar. Peter Duesberg was there, Professor Robert Root-Bernstein of Michigan State University (author of the book *Rethinking AIDS*),[1] Professor Fritz Ulmer from Wuppertal University (mathematician and AIDS doubter), biophysicist Eleni Eleopulos from the Royal Hospital, Perth, Western Australia (author of several important scientific papers challenging the role and identity of HIV), Professor Gordon Stewart, John Lauritsen, Celia Farber and many other European and American delegates.

The conference was called 'AIDS: A Different View' and its organizer, Martien Brands, joined us that evening to check out 'how far we were all going to go' and what Duesberg was going to say about the politically hot subject of 'safer sex' and clean needles campaigns. This was to become a big issue at the end of the conference. But Brands soon realized that there was no controlling this unruly mob, happy at last to be in each others' company after so many years of being slapped down.

The walk in the morning after breakfast along the canalside, reflecting the blue skies and hip-gabled roofs of the grand red brick houses, was beautiful and allowed me time to think over the series of important events that had taken place in the lead-up to this conference. For example, just two weeks before the conference, there had been Neville Hodgkinson's article in the *Sunday Times*, encouraged by the then editor Andrew Neil. It had caused shock waves as the first major piece of journalism in a UK national newspaper to challenge the virus/AIDS hypothesis. It was the first of a series of articles that were immensely important in raising the profile of the dissident debate both in the UK and worldwide. Hodgkinson's first article was extensive, but one quotation from Harvey Bialy had stuck in my mind. In his capacity as editor of *Reappraising AIDS*, the journal of the Group for the Scientific Reappraisal of the HIV/AIDS hypothesis, he told Hodgkinson, 'The virus theory has produced nothing. Efforts based on this approach have had three results: a vaccine that doesn't exist; AZT, which is iatrogenic genocide; and condom use, which is common sense.'[2]

Just three days before the conference opened William Leith wrote an article in the *Independent on Sunday* called 'New Theories, Old Prejudices', describing Peter Duesberg's and Luc Montagnier's positions on HIV and AIDS:

A group of scientists discover something new, something unorthodox, and what happens? The scientific establishment disowns them. ... This has been happening since history began. For example, in 1859, a Cambridge scientist wrote on the eve of the publication of a new book: 'Although I am fully convinced of the truth of the views given in this volume ... I by no means expect to convince experienced naturalists whose minds are stocked with a multitude of facts all viewed, during a long course of years, from a point of view directly opposite to mine.' The scientist was Charles Darwin.

Why do people react so badly to new scientific discoveries? Try to imagine what it's like: there you are, a scientist going about your business perfectly happily, using your old theories and getting along fine. And then somebody comes up with a genuinely new theory. You can't just add it to your old theory. It replaces the old theory. The two cannot coexist. ... As Max Planck wrote: 'A new scientific truth does not triumph by convincing its opponents and making them see the light, but rather because its opponents eventually die and a new generation grows up that is familiar with it.'

Is this what we are seeing now? Are Duesberg and Montagnier a latter-day Darwin or Copernicus? If their theories are correct the whole AIDS culture would be turned on its head. If HIV is not necessary or a sufficient cause of AIDS, then the multimillion pound HIV vaccine industry, is a waste of money. The HIV testing industry, also worth millions of pounds, is a red herring ... there are serious implications for AIDS charities. People might be less compassionate. Government funding might be harder to justify to the voter.[3]

On the following day *The Times* published a lead article called 'AIDS and Truth'; 'AIDS is not a widespread killer. ... Peter Duesberg is no crank,' it said. 'So hysterical has been the reaction to Professor Duesberg as to drive him and any who follow his line of reasoning into virtual ostracism, recalling the fate of Galileo before the Inquisition.' The article ends by saying:

Vested interest should always have a question mark raised over it, not least when it seeks to stamp on efforts of scientists who sincerely believe otherwise. AIDS research, like all scientific discovery, should start not with dogma but with scepticism. ... They should welcome sceptics with open arms, offer them equal riches, test every thesis in the fire of argument and honestly accept the outcome.[4]

With media attention such as this as our backcloth, we thought at last the day of enlightenment had come. And there were more. In the same

1. Professor Peter Duesberg, of the University of California at Berkeley, has for many years challenged the position that AIDS is an infectious condition caused by HIV. His calls for research and funding into other possible explanations for AIDS, including long-term recreational and intravenous drug abuse, have met with stiff resistance from commercial, academic and activist groups for whom the HIV-AIDS hypothesis has become an unchallenged truth.

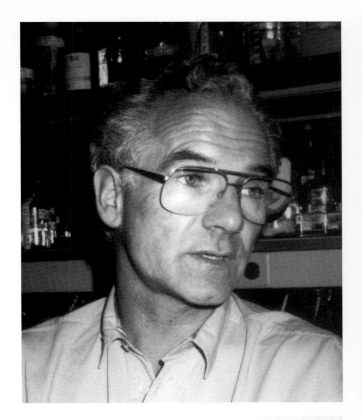

2. Dr Robert Gallo, currently head of the Institute of Human Virology in Maryland, has helped to define the standard orthodoxy on HIV and AIDS yet his research methods have been strongly criticised by three US Government inquiries. His claim to have been the first to isolate the retro-virus HIV has been discredited, though the commercial exploitation of his patented HIV test has fed the proposition that HIV inevitably leads to AIDS.

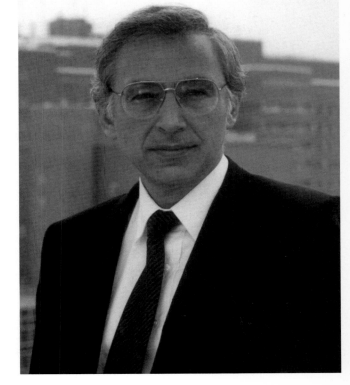

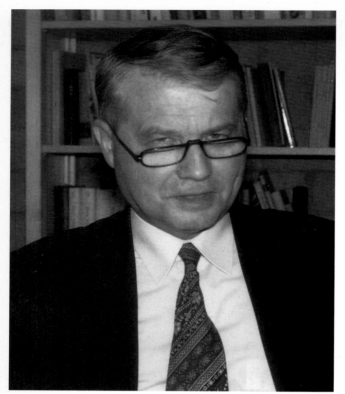

3. Dr Luc Montagnier, of the Pasteur Institute in France, was the first to claim identification of the retro-virus HIV which has led inexorably to the linking of HIV with AIDS. Over the years Montagnier has pointed out that HIV alone cannot cause AIDS without co-factors, giving comfort to some dissidents that even the discoverer of HIV soft pedals on categorical claims for its relation with AIDS.

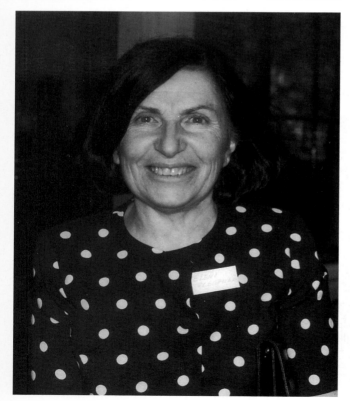

4. Eleni Eleopulos, bio-physicist from Perth, Western Australia, has led a research team which criticizes the way HIV is claimed to have been isolated and identified. She points to anomalies in HIV test results which indicate that HIV has been wrongly identified and may not exist at all.

5. RIGHT. John Lauritsen, writer and journalist, has devoted his recent career to tracking the public debate on AIDS, while attempting to communicate to the public-at-large the growing scepticism of many in the scientific community towards the orthodox explanations of the HIV-AIDS phenomenon.

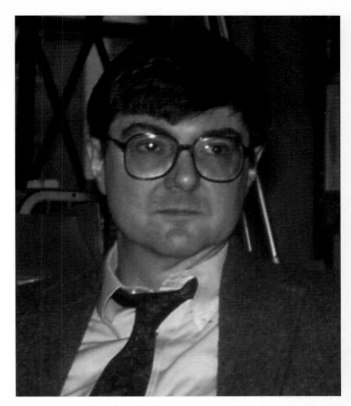

6. BELOW. Dr Harvey Bialy, Science Editor of *Bio/Technology*, with TB specialist Dr Martin Okot-Nwang and his field worker Joseph Nakibali, in Kampala. Bialy has attempted to bring to a wider public the likelihood that "AIDS deaths" in Africa are caused by poverty-linked diseases like TB, whose deadliness is massively exacerbated when misleadingly diagnosed HIV-positives are often denied conventional treatment for their well-known afflictions.

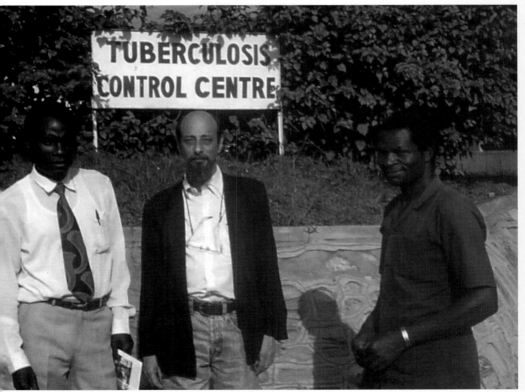

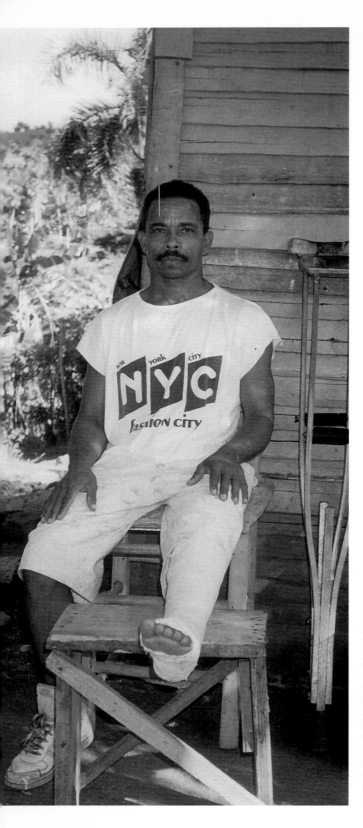

7. Hector Severino, a hotel worker in the Dominican Republic, was diagnosed HIV-positive after a motorcycle accident. Because he was HIV-positive he was denied surgery and has remained disabled. His distraught wife committed suicide, he lost his job and his life was ruined. Two years later he was diagnosed negative on two separate occasions. Severino's case highlights the intrinsic difficulty of HIV tests, where results may be affected by different factors on different occasions.

issue of *The Times*, Charles Bremner filled a whole page with his profile of Duesberg, 'Cast out for an AIDS heresy.'[5]

His extensive article covered both personal and scientific details of Duesberg's life. He mentioned the Gallo–Duesberg feud and the fact that Gallo was described by friends as not being able to discuss the Duesberg hypothesis 'without shrieking'. Bremner also focused on Duesberg's scathing remarks about the repeated revisions of the estimated latency period for developing AIDS.

At first the experts talked of months from infection. Now they said 50 per cent were expected to contract the disease within a decade. 'It's like moving the goal posts, or, in the middle of Wimbledon, you keep raising the net because you're losing', says the professor with one of the metaphors that make him eminently quotable and infuriate the critics who accuse him of playing to the media.

The article ended by describing Duesberg's view that:

The surge in AIDS-type diseases is a direct consequence of the abuse to the human system from the self-administration of toxic drugs such as heroin, nitrites, cocaine, amphetamines and the rest of the armoury of the modern age. The link to homosexuality sprang from the explosion of drug consumption in the wild free-for-all of gay liberation in the 1970s, he says. Yet no studies have investigated the long-term effects of psychoactive drugs on animals comparable with the time periods and dosages used by AIDS patients. 'It's very testable what I'm saying. Why don't we test street drugs and see what it does to the immune system?'

This is how Professor Duesberg arrives at his conclusion that safe sex and clean needles in themselves do nothing to halt the spread of AIDS, a view that incites apoplexy among AIDS workers.

Back at the conference, things began to hot up fairly swiftly. Luc Montagnier set the ball rolling by making a 45-minute speech. It was highly orthodox and had nothing new to say. Montagnier was obviously nervous. Having agreed to come to the conference he now found himself surrounded by dissidents and did not want to be too closely identified with them. His position on HIV as the sole cause of AIDS was ambivalent. He may have regretted some of the things he said to us (in our interview for *The AIDS Catch*) in his enthusiasm to be the first to discover co-factors for HIV. Unfortunately, his mycoplasma theory had come to nothing. Throughout the conference he wanted to make it absolutely clear that although he was on record as saying HIV might not be the sole cause of AIDS, he had definitely not abandoned HIV and left the orthodox camp. He also spoke strongly in favour of AZT.

At this point an element of cold feet began to affect the conference organizers. They did not want to be seen to be hand in glove with the dissidents, so when Duesberg stood up to speak they had decided to allow him only 30 minutes. This was Duesberg's great moment, but his delivery was nervous and rushed. Half way through his detailed speech filled with slides to back up his evidence, he was given windup signals. He protested but to no avail and was cut off in mid flow. Nevertheless, he received a standing ovation from the auditorium and his most important points were reported fairly by Nigel Hawkes in *The Times*.[6]

Then it was Professor Gordon Stewart's turn to set the cat among the pigeons. He predicted that there would be no heterosexual AIDS epidemic in Britain or North America. He said that after 11 years' experience of the spread of AIDS there was no justification for alarmist campaigns saying that everyone was at risk. The number of women infected with AIDS outside the high risk groups was very small. On the basis of this evidence it could not be maintained that there was or would be a heterosexual epidemic. Dr Joe Sonnabend also spoke out strongly about the 'criminal' suppression of research possibilities other than HIV. He said this tragedy had been brought about by the AIDS research establishment and that this distortion of the truth 'may have caused thousands of people to suffer and die'.[7]

During this time, our own production team had been contracted to make a programme for Thames TV's flagship current affairs programme *This Week* based around the Amsterdam conference and focusing on whether or not heterosexuals were in fact at risk of contracting AIDS through straight sex. But once again the heavy hand of opposition intervened. The week before Amsterdam and literally days before we were to begin the shoot, Paul Woolwich, editor of *This Week*, pulled out of his commitment to a programme. His letter intoned:

Both the Department of Health and the Terrence Higgins Trust have told This Week *in no uncertain terms that they fundamentally mistrust you. . . . They would have no problem whatever if* This Week *was doing the programme without Meditel's involvement. Both have cited the BCC adjudication in which your company was judged to have unfairly misrepresented the views of several establishment scientists. Their press officers said it was unlikely they would want to put anyone up for the programme but at least were prepared to give* This Week *a hearing.*

Woolwich went on to say, 'I am no longer convinced we would be able to produce a balanced programme on a controversial issue and it would be journalistically irresponsible of me to proceed any further.'[8] So much for independence in the media. But fortunately we were not entirely muzzled. We had also been commissioned to produce conference reports by Italian producer Stefano Gentiloni at RAI 2, and by Joanne Sawicki at Sky News.

We were thus able to corner Luc Montagnier. To our surprise, he edged ever closer to discrediting HIV as an inevitable AIDS factor. Although he still believed that HIV was necessary for the development of AIDS, he openly admitted that not everyone with HIV would progress to AIDS. He said, 'We are seeing people who have been infected for 9 to 10 years or more – 10 to 12 years, and they are still in good shape. Their immune system is still good. And it is unlikely those people will come down with AIDS later.'[9]

Professor Robert Root-Bernstein, whose rigorous research at Michigan State University into alternative hypotheses on the cause of AIDS had recently completed a search in the literature on prostitutes with alleged HIV/AIDS, was forceful in expressing his doubts about the risk of heterosexual transmission of AIDS:

There have been dozens of studies worldwide on whether female prostitutes develop either HIV or AIDS and every single one of these studies, whether in Europe or the United States has shown definitively that female prostitutes who do get HIV or who develop AIDS are, almost without exception – there are a few exceptions – intravenous drug abusers. If they don't use drugs, they don't get HIV and they don't get AIDS – and they are seeing the same clientele.[10]

Root-Bernstein went on to express anger at the way scientific research has locked itself in for so long to the single theory that HIV is the cause of AIDS.

The anger comes when I think about the people who are dying. Because this is not a question of simply pushing through the research to convince other scientists. This is a question that every month that goes by, we have several hundred or thousands of people who died who might have been able to be helped, if only we'd gotten the research done earlier, or convinced more people to move in this direction.[11]

HIV and Laboratory Contamination

While driving with Montagnier on the Schiphol airport road I had taken the opportunity to question him on his response to one of the scandalous side-shows of the HIV-AIDS saga. Was he the only original source of the accepted HIV virus isolate? Could it be that the virus isolate claimed to have been discovered independently in the UK was also a contaminant of Montagnier's LAV virus, just like Gallo's claims to have isolated HIV in the USA had been no more than an LAV contaminant? Millions of pounds were at stake and the matter is still unresolved.

For years Duesberg had been telling us that the so-called HIV isolates leading to separate patents were in fact the one and only same LAV from Montagnier's lab (namely the Gallo/Montagnier dispute) which, when shared out, as was common practice, had contaminated cell cultures in the host laboratories. Contamination is not at all unusual. It had occurred in Myron Essex's laboratory at Harvard, when he claimed he had found new strains of HIV isolate from an African woman and from an African green monkey. It all turned out to be simple laboratory contamination by the familiar SIV (simian immuno-deficiency virus) from some local zoo monkeys. Contamination of cell cultures can occur via glassware or by virus particles in aerosol drop-lets entering the atmosphere of hoods used to manipulate cultures. Even small amounts of a contaminating virus can take over a new isolate and dominate it.[12]

In the UK, a British team of virologists led by Robin Weiss and Richard Tedder claimed they had isolated their own, different strain of HIV from a patient at the Royal Marsden Hospital. They called it CBL-1 (after the Chester Beatty Laboratory where Weiss was the director) and filed a patent for the test kit in 1986. The patent is held by the Institute of Cancer Research and is licensed to the Wellcome Foun-dation. Until 1991, the main test kit used in the UK to screen blood was based on this isolate. It won the Queen's Award for Technology in 1987. By 1990, Wellcome had sold several million of these tests at about £1 each.

In January 1991 Steve Connor wrote a carefully researched piece in the *Independent on Sunday*, 'Million pound row over AIDS test'. His opening paragraph says it all, 'A cancer charity and British pharma-ceutical company face having to pay millions of pounds to a French research institute [Montagnier's Pasteur Institute] because of a pos-sible patent dispute over the NHS blood test for AIDS.' Connor went on to the nub of the matter: 'The researchers who invented the blood test now believe that they may not have made a new discovery. Because of a laboratory mix-up, they fear they used a discovery from the Pasteur Institute in Paris, contravening a written agreement between the British and French Institutes.'[13]

Weiss apparently claimed to have made all the necessary checks on his isolate, but his findings had been 'muzzled' by the Cancer Institute (the patent holders) and Wellcome (the licensees). A week after Connor's article, Robin Weiss confirmed in *Nature* the close likeness between his isolate and Montagnier's. He admitted that both cultures were being used in his laboratory at the same time and said, 'I cannot exclude the possibility of cross-contamination'.[14]

The implications of this are enormous. After reopening his dispute with Gallo in the USA in 1991* and demanding higher compensation for what he claimed to be Gallo's appropriation of his virus, Montagnier could now turn his guns on the UK and claim millions of pounds back from the UK 'isolate' revenues going into the pockets of Wellcome, Weiss, Tedder and the NHS. So, whether mistakenly or not, it was quite likely that Weiss had called Montagnier's virus his own. According to John Maddox, 'Weiss did the honourable thing by writing to explain his mistake,'[15] but it would have been more honourable if he could have explained his mistake before, not after, Steve Connor wrote about it in the *Independent on Sunday*. It would have been even more honourable if he had admitted having withheld information about CBL-1 for three years during which he held a patent for it together with the Wellcome Foundation.

Now, back in the taxi with Montagnier in Amsterdam, I wanted to find out how he felt about the whole affair and whether he would take any action against the UK. The rumour was that as soon as the Pasteur Institute had finally sorted out the US situation with Gallo it would start proceedings in the UK. As we were driving on the Schiphol highway I told Montagnier that we had been following the Weiss/CBL-1 situation closely. In the light of Weiss's admission in *Nature*, was he going to turn his guns on the UK? He seemed taken aback at first and furrowed his brow. Then he smiled enigmatically and said, 'Robin Weiss is working at the Pasteur Institute just now. Perhaps I will take a walk down the corridor and have a talk with him.'

It is crucial that the matter of the Weiss and Gallo isolates be resolved and not simply for reasons of retribution or financial gain. HIV has, until now, never truly been isolated. It is only identified through complex cell culturing and sequencing in the laboratory, constantly at the risk of contamination, which produce a series of antibodies to proteins said to be HIV specific (that is, said to show up if HIV is present). But, as we shall see later, if the entire HIV edifice is based on the same isolate (Montagnier's) and the basis for testing for it

---

* In July 1994, the Americans agreed to give the Pasteur Institute a greater royalty share of the remaining life of the patent for the Gallo/NIH AIDS test. This was regarded by the Pasteur Institute as official recognition that the virus was isolated in its laboratories in 1983 (*Newsweek*, 25 July 1994).

depends on laboratory artefacts produced by the manipulation of cell cultures and sequences, then this could cast doubt on the very identification and even existence of HIV itself (see Chapter 14).

Backlash from the AIDS Barons

The Amsterdam conference, in essence, was preaching to the converted in that little church. It may have gained a few converts, but it in fact threw up whole new waves of antagonisms. The medical establishment's reaction was dramatic. The MRC's Dr D. A. Rees produced a steaming press release on 15 May, the day after the conference began, called 'Careless talk costs lives'. He opened with:

An epidemic of irresponsible and inaccurate media reports has emerged, centred around an 'alternative' AIDS conference in Amsterdam. These reports publicize the claims of Professor Peter Duesberg that HIV does not cause AIDS. They quote him as saying that AIDS is 'not an infectious disease and it's not a sexually transmitted disease'. They give newspaper space and air time to his statements that safe sex has not prevented a single case of AIDS. And they broadcast his view that the drug AZT is 'AIDS by prescription'. These statements represent a lethal cocktail of untruth and ignorance. . . . To suggest, as Duesberg does, that safer sex is useless in the fight against AIDS is an irresponsibility bordering on the criminal.[16]

There had been a crucial difference of opinion between the Duesberg and Sonnabend factions at the conference on the issue of safe sex. Sonnabend and his group, including Michael Callen, questioned HIV as the cause of AIDS and believed that multiple sexually transmitted infections could undermine the immune system and cause the AIDS syndrome. They were therefore committed to the 'safer sex' campaigns (which they claimed to have started) and the use of condoms, and were keen to obtain Duesberg's endorsement.

Duesberg believes that the body is only overwhelmed by infection *after* the immune system has been broken down by the toxic assault of drugs (intravenous and other recreational drugs as well as some medical ones) and other immune-suppressant factors like blood transfusions and the injection of clotting Factor VIII by haemophiliacs. This breakdown then allowed opportunistic infections to take over the undefended body. Put simply, the breakdown of the immune system is caused by toxic factors, not infectious ones. Although maintaining that condoms were important in avoiding sexually transmitted diseases and unwanted pregnancies, it was Duesberg's view that safe sex had not prevented a single case of AIDS, and that by concentrating exclusively on safe sex and clean needles as preventions against AIDS, people were being lulled into a false sense of security, which in Duesberg's view was utterly misguided and wrong. There was deadlock between the two factions.

The conference ended with acrimonious exchanges. However, all week the key arguments challenging HIV as the cause of AIDS had been telexed, faxed and printed out around the world. When summed up by Lauritsen a great deal of good was gained from this gathering. 'The genie is out of the bottle in Europe,' he wrote, 'and the "AIDS" orthodoxies will never be the same. ... Millions of people are now aware that important scientists, armed with powerful arguments, dispute the official dogma that AIDS is a single disease entity caused solely by a retrovirus called the "Human immunodeficiency virus (HIV)".'[17]

The immediate reaction in the UK following the conference was depressingly predictable. Dr Kenneth Calman, the Department of Health's Chief Medical Officer, said that Duesberg's views 'have been extensively discussed and refuted. ... My view, supported by the great majority of medical and scientific opinion, is that the evidence that HIV causes AIDS is overwhelming.' However, towards the end of his piece Calman writes, 'We have much more to learn about HIV and AIDS. We do not yet fully understand the exact process by which HIV infection progresses to AIDS or why the disease does not develop at the same rate in everyone infected. There is a need for more research. This does not change the crucial conclusion that HIV causes AIDS.'[18]

The reaction in the medical and science journals after the conference was, on the whole, hostile. On 23 May, the *Lancet* published an article by Jaap Goudsmit, a Dutch scientist at the conference who, together with Roel Coutinho and Frank Miedema, had been most hostile to the Duesberg hypothesis. Coutinho and Miedema had openly shouted Duesberg down, even pulling faces at him. One evening when the sessions had ended Duesberg was invited to join Coutinho, Miedema and others in an upstairs room in the church for an impromptu discussion. It turned into an attack on Duesberg in which he was simply shouted at for being wrong. When Duesberg pointed out the absurdity of a situation where no other retrovirus had ever been shown to cause disease in man, that this one (HIV) was supposed not only to cause disease, but to kill you ten years on, they simply said, 'Well, this one does.'[19]

Gaudsmit was given two full-length columns in the *Lancet* to dismiss Duesberg's arguments with no space offered for a reply from Duesberg. For the editor of the *Lancet* to decide to allow Goudsmit, a committed member of the AIDS establishment, to sum up the whole conference, with not an inch of space allowed any of the eminent dissident scientists there, seemed very wrong. Besides, to choose Goudsmit, of all people, was a grave error indeed. We had learned at the conference that a year earlier, Goudsmit's own research into HIV had come under a very large cloud. He and his colleague Henck Buck published a claim that they had found a way of blocking the infectivity of HIV. Their work was submitted to four separate university investigations which eventually demolished all the claims made in their paper. In an article in *Science*, Felix Eijgenraam described how Buck was relieved of his duties as dean of faculty and chairman at Eindhoven Technical University's department of organic chemistry, and how the University of Amsterdam Medical Faculty found Goudsmit guilty of making unjustifiable claims, of biased selection of data and misleading presentation of facts.[20] When I wrote a letter to the *Lancet* to point out Goudsmit's recent experience, deputy editor David Sharp after a month replied that the *Lancet* 'will not be able to find room for it. In the face of fierce competition it just failed to find a place.'[21]

The repeated suppression of any information that might be critical of the AIDS establishment was no longer a surprise to me. More was to come. Following the indignation of Professors Klug and Perutz at Cambridge after our programme *The AIDS Catch*, the events in Amsterdam proved too much for them yet again. So, together with another two scientists, Nobel Laureate, Cesar Milstein and Abraham Karpas, they wrote in high dudgeon to the *Independent*:

Unfortunately, the prominence given to Duesberg's views two years ago on a Channel 4 television programme (Dispatches, 13 June 1990), and now reinforced in the Press in connection with the recent so-called Alternative AIDS conference in Amsterdam, can only serve to accelerate the spread of the virus.

Since all medical and scientific evidence indicates beyond any doubt that HIV is the cause of AIDS, we hope that your newspaper will continue to educate the public as long as it continues to be necessary to do so.[22]

I knew of the strong commitments to the HIV hypothesis of three of the signatories (Klug, Perutz and Karpas). Abraham Karpas himself had told us in a filmed interview that he had developed his own HIV isolate and test kit, that a Japanese company was interested and that it had been submitted to the NHS for treatment of AIDS patients. I also knew that Klug and Perutz were involved in ongoing HIV research at the Cambridge MRC laboratories. We had counted four major HIV-based projects there, including HIV-1 regulatory proteins, anti-HIV agents, and nucleoside HIV-antiviral agents. (We later discovered through Labour MP George Galloway's series of hard hitting questions on AZT and AIDS tabled in the House of Commons in May 1993, that between 1989 and 1993 the government had provided a total of £68 million to the MRC for HIV and AIDS research.)[23]

We decided to respond to the accusations in the *Independent*. An accompanying article in the *Independent* by Steve Connor, published together with the letter from the Cambridge group of scientists, had specifically attacked us, *The Times* and the *Sunday Times* for our reporting on the Amsterdam conference. So, having discussed the matter with the then editor of *The Times*, Simon Jenkins, I wrote two letters to the editor of the *Independent*, Andreas Whittam Smith, in our defence. The letter suggested that it would have been fairer if the interests of the signatories had been declared. Both letters were rejected for publication.[24]

Jenkins agreed that I should ask Whittam Smith to take the matter to his newspaper's ombudsman, Sir Gordon Downey, later to become parliamentary commissioner for standards. Sir Gordon's reply was brief: 'Your suggestion that, because of their research in the field, the signatories to the letter published on 20 May should "declare an interest" is, I think unworthy. Had they no direct experience, their qualifications for commenting would have been much reduced."[25] However, Jenkins did not leave it at that. He wrote a private letter to Whittam Smith expressing his concern that in areas of medical research, where large sums of government money are involved, often linked with pharmaceutical companies, editors should be careful to ask for interests to be declared.[26]

It is understandable that anyone who is closely involved with a subject should wish to air their expertise and the fact that they may be receiving financial reward for their work in that particular field in no way impugns their integrity or disqualifies them from being heard. The important thing is that their interests be declared and known. Our frustration stemmed from the fact that anyone from the orthodoxy could get a hearing or their letters published while ours were rejected. And if we requested that our critics' links, whether financial or professional, to HIV funded research be declared, we were ignored.

Chapter 10

'AIDS and Africa'

Rakai village, Uganda: The Epicentre of AIDS?

Human beings are full of retroviruses, and neither HIV nor any other retrovirus by itself poses any kind of threat. Which is not to say that there is no such thing as AIDS – only that HIV doesn't cause it.

(Dr Kary Mullis, Nobel prize winner, Chemistry, 1993)[1]

Something on the floor stirred under the light cotton blanket. We had walked out of the intense sunlight in the village square into the darkness of a small mud and thatch house. There lay Najemba. Thin as a stick, she tried with difficulty to sit up. Her eyes were deeply sad as she looked up at us helplessly. Our guide Yassin Balinda translated quickly and quietly from Najemba's native Luganda language. 'I can't walk,' she said. 'You see, it's my legs.' She pulled back the blanket and we saw the skin infection on her legs. Some areas were raw and inflamed, others had huge scabs. Najemba's brother Gerald told us that the whole village believed Najemba had AIDS. But she had never seen a doctor and she had never had a blood test. 'Slim (AIDS) is a formula for everything here,' said Gerald. 'When somebody dies we call it slim.' Gerald explained how, because he had to feed his wife and young children, he often didn't have enough food to go round for Najemba, but a while back he had managed to get some antibiotics for Najemba's skin infection. It had cleared up, but now the village hospital had started charging for the WHO medicines and he could not afford them.

I was travelling with journalist Celia Farber. We both fumbled in our purses and found what little money we had to buy her a course of antibiotics. I had made up my mind that I would be coming back to the village in a few months' time with our film crew, but I did not expect to see Najemba alive again.

Rakai village had not been on our itinerary authorized by Uganda's Ministry of Health, but we made an unauthorized visit to find out what was happening in this area the world had named the epicentre of AIDS. Although the village looked neglected, this was no ghost town. There were men, women and children milling about in the dusty main street and in the square. We made our way to a small bar serving beer and soft drinks. Celia decided to walk into the village square and that was where she had met Gerald, who eventually led us to Najemba. Meanwhile, I had stayed on at the bar and struck up a conversation with some Methodist charity workers who were setting up a school in the village. 'The problem,' said one of them, 'is not so much AIDS, it's the fact that the people here just don't have enough to eat. They are dying of malnutrition.'

When I related this story to friends back home, they would say. 'But how could they be dying of hunger? Look at your photographs, they show green fields, trees and fertile earth? Surely they could live off the land?' This is a classic misunderstanding. How can they live off the land if they have no seed whatsoever, not a single hoe between them and, to avoid starving, have eaten last year's seed crop? The desperate nutritional state of people living in the Rakai had been recognized only the week before, by Uganda's president himself, Yoweri Musseveni. His speech describing the need for food supplies and agricultural aid had been headline news in the papers.

Plans for our research trip had started several months earlier when David Lloyd at Channel 4 had suggested we focus our AIDS research efforts on Africa. He then agreed to give us development money for our proposed film *AIDS and Africa*. Lloyd wanted us to take with us a doctor or scientist as a Western observer. I chose Dr Harvey Bialy, scientific editor of *Bio/Technology*, who had worked for many years in Africa as a tropical diseases expert. Bialy had for some time been concerned about the way AIDS was being blamed on Africa and in particular about the increasing number of sloppily researched papers written by Western AIDS researchers about the sub-Saharan continent.

As early as 1988, in an interview with Drew Hopkins for *City Week*, Bialy said:

There is no scientific literature about AIDS in Africa. It is 100 per cent ad hominem, anecdotal trash. There is scarcely a single paper of any substance that has come out of the so-called epidemic of AIDS in Africa. I had thought for a long time that what was being classified as AIDS in Africa, which was a completely different syndrome of diseases than what was being called AIDS in the West, was in fact nothing more than a new name for a collection of old diseases. Diseases that are called AIDS are classical African diseases in populations that have for a very long time been subject to these infections. When that is readjusted in terms of terribly, terribly bad sero-epidemiology, in regard to the so-called AIDS virus, the picture becomes a very grim one, at least a statistically grim one. The whole notion of African AIDS is sick to begin with. Why is there such a thing as African AIDS? Do we have American AIDS, Asian AIDS, French AIDS?[2]

At this time Drs Anton Geser and Glen Burbaker had released the manuscript of their paper called 'AIDS in Africa: an alternative hypothesis'. The paper's opening paragraph said:

The present paper proposes an alternative hypothesis according to which AIDS is not a new disease in Africa (nor indeed anywhere), and HIV not the cause of the syndrome, but merely a passenger virus which flourishes more freely in immunodepressed hosts. This new hypothesis is applied to the AIDS problem in Africa and certain consequences of the alternative views are pointed out, of which the most important is that the devastating AIDS epidemic, now being predicted in Africa, will not occur.[3]

The paper notes that even after the introduction of broader criteria for the diagnosis of AIDS in Africa, like 'slim disease' and the agreed WHO Bangui clinical case definition whereby a combination of symptoms like fever for a month, diarrhoea and a dry cough could lead to a confirmed AIDS diagnosis, the number of actual AIDS cases in Africa remained low. Geser and Burbaker continued, 'In five countries with the highest case reporting the accumulated figures by mid-1987 were as follows: Uganda 1138, Tanzania 1130, Rwanda 705, Kenya 625, and Zaire 335.'

I planned a research trip that took in the countries where most foreign aid money had been granted for AIDS research. This took Bialy, Farber (who was writing a feature on AIDS)[4] and myself first to the Ivory Coast, and then eastwards to Uganda, Tanzania and Kenya. In each country we visited hospitals and laboratories and spoke to scientists, doctors, patients and health workers, some who were committed to the virus/AIDS hypothesis and a surprising number who were not. We were to draw heavily on Harvey Bialy's extensive experience in Africa, his credentials as a molecular biologist and his impressions of the current AIDS picture after our wide ranging research trip together. This is how he later set the tone for our film: 'From both my literature review and my personal experience over most of the so-called AIDS centres in Africa, I can find no believable, persuasive evidence that Africa is in the midst of a new epidemic of infectious immunodeficiency.'[5] I retraced my steps later when I returned with our film crew, but another highlight of our research trip is worth recording.

Philippe Krynen, working in Bukoba, Tanzania for a French charity called Partage, had faxed our hotel in Kampala to say we should meet him at the Ugandan border with Tanzania. 'It's too difficult to get the car across,' wrote Krynen, 'so leave your car and walk through into no-man's land where there is one tree. I shall be standing under it,' he wrote. And so he was, blue jeans, cowboy boots and open-necked shirt, a lithe, restless man, with sharp determined features and an inexhaustible energy. Krynen was furious at the way AIDS figures were being distorted and exaggerated in his area around Lake Victoria, and had succeeded in getting a whole village in his project area to volunteer to be tested in order to 'get to the truth'. He had brought some members of his team with him so we adjourned to a tiny room where they sold beer and soft drinks, and talked for hours about his work, and about the anger he felt at the way his communities were becoming demoralized and physically undermined because of the AIDS plague terror campaigns. It was at this meeting that Krynen told us he would be announcing the results of his own HIV survey at the forthcoming African international AIDS conference in Yaounde, Cameroon. We agreed to meet there and film his announcement.

Why Did Africa Get the Blame for AIDS?

By the mid-1980s it had become widely accepted that AIDS originated in Africa. It was Dr Kevin de Cock from the Institute of Hygiene and Tropical Medicine who set the ball rolling by suggesting that AIDS was an 'old disease from Africa'.[6] Next Robert Gallo, in the company of his colleague Max Essex stepped in and put forward the monkey hypothesis – that an African green monkey virus jumped species infecting humans and subsequently spread throughout the world.[7] Then, Dr Anthony Pinching at St Mary's Hospital, London threw in the notion that people in central Africa had a genetic predisposition to infection with HIV.[8] Later on, Cambridge scientist, Abraham Karpas, drew attention to an obscure anthropological work in which the author claimed that it was a local custom near the shores of Lake Victoria for men and women to inoculate themselves in the loins with monkey blood as an aphrodisiac.[9] As late as 1992, when most scientists had quietly dropped the African connection, Professor Roy Anderson at Imperial College, London was still stating that: 'The AIDS virus almost certainly evolved in Africa.'[10]

These theories had absolutely no basis in science. They were pieces of pure speculation from 'the keepers of wisdom', but they did untold damage to Africa and its people. In the end, Pinching admitted that his theory was based on erroneous data.[11] The monkey theory was thrown out of the window when Japanese molecular biologists discovered that the green monkey virus (SIV) differed by more than 50 per cent when compared with HIV. They concluded there was no genetic relationship between the human and the monkey virus.[12] Dr Alan Cantwell, writing for the *New African* says:

The African origin of AIDS has been debunked by several epidemiological studies. When a team of scientists led by J. W. Carswell tested the blood of old, sexually inactive people living in geriatric homes in the Ugandan capital Kampala ... the team discovered that none of the elderly people tested positive for HIV *antibodies. This 1986 study concluded that the virus had not been around Uganda for a long time.*[13]

Another important study by Professor G. Hunsmann, head of virology and immunology at Göttingen University, was able to make use of more than 6000 frozen and stored serum samples from all over central Africa. The study concludes, 'fewer than one in 1000 subjects were seropositive for AIDS at the time of sampling before 1985 and do not support the hypothesis of the disease originating in Africa.'[14] Hunsmann's findings of 0.1 per cent HIV positivity in the general population of Africa was very low indeed. It was even lower than the estimated figures for HIV positive people in the USA at the time, which was between 0.2 and 3 per cent of the population.

Two books cover this territory well, tackling both scientific issues and the racist attitudes involved in the association of AIDS with Africa – *What is AIDS?* by Dr Felix Konotey-Ahulu[15] and *AIDS, Africa and Racism* by Richard and Rosalind Chirimuuta.[16] Konotey-Ahulu had been concerned about false reporting on AIDS in Africa for some time. After a trip through Africa in 1987, he wrote in the *Lancet*: '"Why do the world's media appear to have conspired with some scientists to become so gratuitously extravagant with the untruth?" – that was the question uppermost in the minds of intelligent Africans and Europeans I met on my tour.'[17] Richard Chirimuuta described how 'blaming Africa' led to a stream of absurd and damaging speculations about 'African behaviour'.

There were many, many examples but one example is that Africans gave their children dead monkeys to play with as toys and there was all this nonsense about how much more promiscuous Africans were than any other humans. I could go on and on. That Africans believe that the only cure for AIDS was to sleep with virgins and this is why AIDS was so widespread in Africa. Most of them were all based on racism or racist preconceptions of Africans. The allegations that Africans were more promiscuous than the rest of the human race were unfounded. They didn't make any sense scientifically. In fact when they sent teams of researchers, sociologists and anthropologists to Africa, they were amazed that Africans were actually much more conservative in their sexual practices.[18]

The knock-on effects of those idle speculations by people like Gallo, Essex, Pinching and Karpas were very serious. They led to the ostracism and isolation of African students on scholarships abroad; they led to a fever of HIV testing in Africa by foreign governments and university project researchers, dipping into wards, taking blood, flying it out and coming up with grossly exaggerated estimates of HIV and AIDS incidence for the country and the continent. They led to the flooding in of money from aid agencies like the UK Overseas Development Agency, the MRC, the European Community, WHO, USAID, the NIH, the Centers for Disease Control and countless non-governmental organizations, which in turn set up testing laboratories or initiated sex education programmes and organized the distribution of condoms.

There have been two disastrous consequences from all this misguided activity. Estimates for HIV seroprevalence and AIDS rocketed out of control, resulting in predictions like those of Professor Roy Anderson at Imperial College, London, of a pandemic that would lead to a decrease in the population and political social disturbances in the continent of Africa.[19] But the most serious after-effect was the gradual neglect of the real killers in Africa – malaria, TB and parasitic infections. There was little or no money left for medication and control of these. The 'condom evangelists' and 'safe sex missionaries', as Charles Geshekter calls them, had won the day, while more and more people were left to die from otherwise treatable diseases through lack of basic medicines.

Geshekter, Professor of African history at the California State University in Chico, encapsulates the situation in the following words:

Africans often die, of 'AIDS-like' symptoms after their systems have been weakened by malaria, tuberculosis, cholera or parasitic infections. Venereal diseases left untreated can also impair anyone's immunity, rendering the victim susceptible to infection.

Calling these deaths AIDS and claiming it is endemic provides tantalizing opportunities for development agencies, academics and bio-medical researchers who clamour for more money and state intervention.

Perpetuating the myth of an 'African AIDS epidemic' caused by sexual promiscuity deepens African dependency on infusions of Western aid for diagnostic tests, high-tech sterilization equipment, medical personnel and drug therapies.

It is the political economy of under-development, not heterosexual intercourse that imperils African lives. Poor harvests, rural poverty, migratory labour systems, urban crowding, ecological degradation and the sadistic violence of civil wars claim far more lives. When essential services for water, power and transport break down, public sanitation deteriorates, and the risks of cholera and dysentery increase. Poverty is the best predictor of AIDS-defining diseases.[20]

Bukoba, Tanzania: AIDS Dissident in the Front Line

The reports and images on television from Africa had been of unremitting horror. The WHO described sub-Saharan Africa as having the highest rates of HIV infection in the world – an estimated one in 40 adults – and predicted that by the end of the century there would be half a million deaths a year. 'More people are dying' was the phrase we always heard. But what we discovered on our research trip was that there is no way of comparing 'then' and 'now' deaths because deaths are not registered in any of the countries we visited. We also knew that the figures for HIV and AIDS were being grossly inflated by international agencies and by corrupt government officials. International agencies were awash with funds for Third World AIDS research and sex education programmes. They wanted to get into African countries, and by the same token many African health officials, keen to draw that money in, were happy to fan the flames of AIDS panic by inflating their estimated AIDS and HIV positive figures.

The vast majority of AIDS cases in Africa were not diagnosed with HIV tests; these were too expensive for general use. AIDS was (and still is) diagnosed through the guidelines laid down by the WHO's Bangui clinical case definition. That is, they were not actually tested for HIV but were diagnosed positive or negative on the basis of a combination of symptoms. This is called presumptive diagnosis. The trouble was that the combination of symptoms required for an AIDS diagnosis (prolonged fever, diarrhoea, dry cough) were indistinguishable from those of old established diseases like TB and malaria.

With the research trip behind us, we returned to shoot in December 1992. Once more Philippe Krynen was waiting for us at the Uganda/Tanzania border. Krynen and his French wife Evelyne lived in a house on a hill high above the town of Bukoba with a magnificent view over Lake Victoria. Next to the house was their small clinic for sick children. Krynen's team provided medical care, schooling and support for children in 15 villages spread over a vast region spanning more than 1000 square miles. So great was the fear of AIDS in this community that Philippe had found it difficult to generate community support for the children. 'How can you ask people who believe they are going to die tomorrow, how can you ask them to look into the future which are the children? They give up, they don't invest. They don't want to work in northern Kagera because they think that they are going to die of AIDS, or to contract it.'[21]

Philippe and Evelyne were convinced that if people found to be HIV positive received the right care and support, they could recover. Exactly this happened with Lucy, one of their young trainees who was an orphan. Lucy became ill with repeated infections and lost more than 20 pounds in weight. She became very withdrawn and everyone thought she had AIDS. Philippe was so worried about her that he took her to the local hospital where he discovered that she had been diagnosed as HIV positive in an unconfirmed screening test. Philippe and his wife decided to support Lucy and help her regain her position in the community. They moved her out of her small hut and built a cement house for her and offered her a more responsible job with better pay. Says Philippe:

And slowly in four or five months time Lucy started to recover, to put on weight. ... And because she put on weight again her friends started to look at her differently, not putting her aside and not being afraid of her, because they started to question if she really had AIDS or not. It is very seldom you see people who have been stigmatized with AIDS, who are not dying a few months later. So Lucy was one of the first persons who, because we didn't support the AIDS tag on her, recovered and was proof to the community that you can recover from such episodes.[22]

In three successive tests Lucy was found to he HIV negative. She is just one example of the mass of flawed HIV statistics that bedevil Africa, and the inaccuracies of testing. Her initial unconfirmed screening test would have been included in the official reported figures for HIV positives. Krynen had decided to conduct his own HIV survey in the region and was to announce the results at a press conference at the forthcoming AIDS conference in Cameroon.

HIV awareness campaigns had led most people in the region to believe they were infected and WHO publications had put the figure at over 60 per cent. Krynen was unconvinced. For one thing, he noticed that the number of so-called AIDS deaths had diminished in his area over the past two years. He decided to get at the facts. First, he asked all his 160 workers if they would volunteer for confirmed HIV tests. He found 5 per cent were positive. Then a whole village of 842 people volunteered. He found 13.8 per cent were positive. These figures are substantially lower than previous estimates for this region of Tanzania. Krynen told us: 'This is the first time in Africa that a whole village has volunteered as a whole to be tested for a deadly disease. The truth has been five times lower than the figures given by the WHO AIDS Control Programme.'[23] Later Harvey Bialy succinctly confirmed Krynen's position:

Some of these tests are so non-specific that 80–90 per cent of the positives that are picked up are false positives. They're reacting to antibodies that are not HIV specific. And when one realizes that these tests are being pushed in a context in which we have to test as many people as possible, the inevitable outcome is that Africa – the figures for numbers of HIV infections in Africa – will become wildly exaggerated and feed into a very, very deadly self-fulfilling prophesy.[24]

HIV Test False Positive Results

A scan through the scientific literature on the subject worldwide showed that cross-reactions could lead to false positives in people with malaria, TB, leprosy, leishmaniasis, lupus, Chagas disease and sleeping sickness.[25] In 1991, seven out of ten blood donors treated with influenza virus vaccine were declared HIV antibody positive, but when further tested proved to be negative.[26] One astonishing example of false positive results is documented in a letter to the *Lancet* from Dr Alexander Voevodin of the Institute of Pulmonology in Moscow. In 1991, in a mass screening operation in Russia, out of 29.4 million tests, 30,000 were found to be false positives with only 66 confirmations.[27]

Confusion surrounding the clinical diagnosis of full-blown AIDS (as opposed to being found to be HIV positive) was also causing problems. In a letter to the *Lancet* from a group of doctors working in Tanzania, Andrew Swai wrote: 'We are concerned lest newly presenting diabetic patients may be mistakenly thought to have AIDS.' Swai described a man with diabetes mellitus who nearly died because the doctor treating him thought he had AIDS and was reluctant to do anything until the results of the HIV test were known. 'In tropical Africa febrile illnesses are frequently attributed to malaria. Now in certain places AIDS is the fashionable diagnosis, made by the public and doctors. Many patients with treatable and curable illnesses may now be condemned without proper assessment. Public and medical education on AIDS should stress that symptoms such as those described are not unique to AIDS.'[28]

Myron Essex himself, a leading member of the group surrounding Robert Gallo nicknamed the Bob Club, initially found a very high incidence of HIV positivity in Zaire. This had to be lowered by 70 per cent when it was shown that in areas where the leprosy bacillus was endemic, cross-reaction was giving a false HIV positive result.[29]

Return to the Rakai: The African Poverty Trap

Once our visit to Bukoba was over, we drove back to Uganda, determined to return to Rakai village to find Najemba. On the way there we stopped off at the town of Kyotera where we had been given some contacts. We had heard that whenever foreign visitors arrived in this area, a carefully orchestrated show was put on. All the children were brought together and encouraged to put their hands up when they were asked if they were orphans. In Uganda, a child is called an orphan if one parent has died. Many children would put their hands up who were real orphans, part-orphans and not orphans at all (for example if their parents had migrated to find work elsewhere, leaving them with their grandparents). These figures would be taken back to the aid agencies as evidence of an adult AIDS epidemic. We met town official, Badru Ssemanda, who was indignant at the way AIDS was being manipulated in his area for nefarious reasons.

People are trying to make a living out of this [AIDS]. They think that if they publicize it and they exaggerate it, they might win sympathy from the international community and will get aid, or rather get assistance. We need assistance but not through bluffing people and saying that people are dying at a rate which is not true.[30]

We then went to inspect the local water supply, a foul-smelling pool next to the effluent from the town drain. When it rained the water became even more contaminated. Many people did not have the energy or the fuel to boil the water before drinking it. We watched children dipping their plastic containers into the water and carrying them off, gracefully balanced on their heads. But these waters were more dangerous than any supposed virus. These waters carried infections and parasites that could gradually destroy even the strongest man's immune system.

We had met up with Ugandan radio journalist Sam Mulondo who told us that when people developed diarrhoea or other infections they would be so terrified it could be AIDS that they got worse and often died. 'People are dying psychologically. ... Somebody gets simple malaria, they fear to go to the doctor because they will be branded as a clinical case of AIDS. ... People are just left at home. They don't go for any treatment whatsoever.'[31]

That evening I was to learn how the ravages of civil war over the preceding decade had left this town and the whole area with no medical or social infrastructure whatsoever. Our driver, Yassin Balinda, told me how he had been a platoon commander in the liberating forces that advanced through this town from Tanzania to overthrow President Idi Amin. He offered to drive me round the town. As we drove past an open-air cinema I was curious to find out why more people were sitting outside the cinema walls than inside. Then I saw a cloud of insects, stunned by the cinema lights, and falling to the ground. The people outside the cinema were eagerly catching them in tin mugs. 'Locusts' said Yassin. 'They are a local delicacy. Very nutritious and tasty when fried.'

In the centre of town Yassin pointed to several cracked and tilted buildings that had received a pummelling with shells. 'We did that,' he said. 'We had to because we thought there were snipers inside. But finally we realized that the whole town was deserted. Everyone had fled into the bush and every single public building, hospital, clinic, and dispensary was abandoned. There was nobody left. It stayed that way for a long time.' The next day as I walked into Rakai village square my heart was beating fast. Would we be able to find Najemba's brother Gerald? Would Najemba be alive? Then we saw Gerald walking towards us. After our greetings I quickly asked 'How is Najemba?' 'She is in the banana grove,' said Gerald. 'I will call her. She is very weak and she has been told to leave her house.' Najemba walked slowly towards us, breathing heavily. She sat down for a while with us and showed us how her leg infections had cleared up with the antibiotics. 'How do you feel now?' I asked. 'I don't feel too bad but what I lack is things to drink.'

Then she told us sadly that she had been evicted from her house in the square because the village thought she had AIDS, and she was in arrears with her rent. She was trying to build herself a little mud hut in the banana grove. We followed her down there and saw that Najemba was building what was to become her tomb. In the damp low-lying banana grove, infested with malaria mosquitoes she had managed to build some mud walls with a scanty palm roofing. We asked her to work out how much some medicines and a year's rent for her old house would be. The total came to £74. We left this in her hands and said goodbye. If Najemba dies her death will be blamed on AIDS, but the real cause of death, in my view, will have been her destitute living conditions and the cruelty and humiliation of her social rejection.

Before leaving Rakai village we drove up to its small rural hospital on the hill. It was completely deserted – no patients, no staff and a large empty ward with dismantled beds leaning against the walls. This was the so-called epicentre of AIDS and there was not an AIDS patient in sight. Then we heard a sound and walked through into a side room where the only patient lay – a four month old baby with malarial convulsions. The family stood round his bed or sat, feet tucked under them, on the floor in a silent tragic frieze. The medicines from the hospital were not working, the baby would need a stronger one, available only in the town, an hour's drive away. Yes, there was a nurse we could speak to but she had gone off to bed. She too had malaria.

I climbed up to a small cottage and a woman came out to greet me who looked very ill indeed. She was Nurse Namuburu Maxensia, the only member of staff at the hospital. I told her who we were and she seemed keen to help us with information. Ill as she was, she came back to the hospital with us where she unlocked a large wooden cupboard door and showed us a stock of drugs supplied free by the WHO's Essential Drugs Programme. These medicines used to be supplied free to the villagers but, under a new plan, a reduced fixed rate was being charged – as if anyone in the village could afford it. So that was why Gerald could no longer get antibiotics to help Najemba. Nurse Maxensia told us that before the new plan had been introduced the hospital was full and there were sometimes 50 outpatients. 'But now we get few,' she said ruefully, 'because they can't afford to pay.'[32]

Melanie Wangler, our production manager, passed the hat around the crew and we scraped up enough money to send the sick baby to town by hired truck. At that moment a man on a motorcycle came up the hill to find out what we were doing. He told Nurse Maxensia that we did not have permission to be there. We thanked her and left quickly, heading for the road to Kampala.

A few miles away from Rakai village, amid the desolation we noticed a neatly clipped hedge surrounding a smart cottage and garden. In the driveway was a gleaming Toyota. 'Who lives there?' I asked Sam Mulondo. 'The American couple who run the Rakai sex counselling programme,' he replied. We drove in and found a young man wearing shorts and a gold earring on the veranda and a young woman inside the house. Both were absorbed with their laptop computers. We exchanged greetings and left quickly. I felt sick. There they were, the 'condom evangelists' safe in their precinct. The 'safe sex missionaries' made occasional sallies with condoms stuffed in the back of their

Toyota, telling the people of Rakai that it was their fault if they got ill because they had made love to somebody new.

Kampala, Uganda:
Are TB and Malaria Being Called AIDS?

The scourge of well-meaning but misguided Westerners redefining Africa's problems and imposing their solutions was well described by Uganda's Minister of Health, Dr James Makumbi:

We have more than 700 non-governmental organizations operating in the AIDS field in Uganda. This raises concern, because a few of them are doing a very good job. But a good number of them, my ministry is not aware of what they are actually doing, and there is no way of evaluating them. Unfortunately, a good number of them do rush in, collect data and go away with it, and the next we hear about it is when it is being printed in journals. And we have not had any input. Some of the work has been done in very limited areas, not reflecting the rest of the country.[33]

As a result of the redefined AIDS problem, coping with malaria, a curable disease, had become seriously neglected with cutbacks in funding for malaria control and medication. In 1992, the budget from the WHO for malaria control was less than $57,000,[34] while funding from all agencies for AIDS was over $6 million.

Mulago Hospital has a long tradition of excellence in tropical medicine. Separated by a few hundred yards from the main six-floor concrete building is a complex of low huts surrounded by a high wire fence. This is Old Mulago TB Hospital. Dr Martin Okot-Nwang, one of Uganda's leading TB specialists, showed me into one of his wards. He was concerned about the way AIDS statistics were being wrongly reported. He accepted that TB cases had increased over the past few years and explained the reason why. 'We have just recently undergone a series of wars in this country, and this has led to a breakdown in our health services. It's not unknown that following war and famine, increases do occur in infectious or communicable diseases, of which TB is one.'[35]

The rise in TB cases in Africa has led some scientists to speculate that

HIV is making people more susceptible to the disease and that TB patients who are HIV positive have a different medical picture – they 'get more infections and die quicker'. However, it is hard to find any evidence for this. What is documented is that flaws in the clinical case definition, that is the combination of symptoms used for diagnosing AIDS without an HIV test, have meant that many TB cases have mistakenly been called AIDS. Okot-Nwang told us:

A patient who has TB and is HIV positive would appear exactly the same as a patient who has TB and is HIV negative. Clinically both patients could present with long fever, both patients present with loss of weight, both patients actually present with a prolonged cough, and in both cases the cough could be equally productive. Therefore, clinically, I cannot differentiate between the two. Even when I look at the blood analyses I may find some similarities between the two groups.

In the past, only extra-pulmonary TB, not TB of the lung (pulmonary TB), was classified as a disease that qualified as AIDS by the US Centers for Disease Control, but lung TB was added to their list in January 1993. I put this to Dr Okot-Nwang. He simply laughed and said, 'I think if they include pulmonary tuberculosis as an AIDS defining case then all the TBs in Africa – almost all the TBs in Africa – will be AIDS.'[36] I left Dr Okot-Nwang with a feeling of dread as his words echoed in my mind. If all TBs in Africa are called AIDS then more and more TB patients will be totally abandoned 'because they are going to die anyway'. Where attempts at treatment are made, we'd be back to that old vicious circle – money for TB will be diverted into sex counselling and condoms – no money left for TB medication.

Yaounde, Cameroon:
African International AIDS Conference

The seventh international African AIDS conference in Yaounde, Cameroon was indeed a grand affair, drawing together all the national and international dignitaries of the AIDS round. Plumed fountains cast a light spray over the chauffeur-driven stretch limousines that wove in and out of the forecourt fetching and carrying ambassadors, UN and WHO officials, 'leading scientists' and pharmaceutical company reps.

Inside, more than 2000 delegates milled around at what can only be described as an 'AIDS bazaar'. Stand upon stand was selling a whole range of HIV test kits, including the quickie dipstick one. AIDS cures were on offer; safe-sex education cartoons; and at a central stand, as young maidens in white T-shirts offered you every size and colour of condom you could ever wish for, a youth in a dark suit held a large carved ebony-coloured penis aloft as he slowly rolled a condom up and down it.

Philippe Krynen had arrived to hold his press conference. The audience in these surroundings of total commitment to the ravages of HIV in Africa was hostile. Nevertheless, he held his own under concerted attacks from WHO officials and the condom evangelist brigade. He reported on the survey he had conducted in his region of Kagera, Tanzania. The number of AIDS deaths in his area had dropped in the past two years, he said, and official estimates for HIV positivity were vastly inflated. Whereas WHO publications had put the figures for HIV positives at 60 per cent, he had found only 5 per cent of his 160 workers were positive. When he tested his whole village (842 volunteers) he found 13.8 per cent were positive.[37]

These figures are higher than estimates for the number of HIV positives in the West, which are below 1 per cent, but substantially lower that previous estimates for this region of Tanzania. The reason for the alleged higher HIV incidence in Africa is because persistent assault of the body's immune defences through disease, malnutrition and dirty water produces raised antibodies that can test false positive on HIV test kits.

In January 1995, I received New Year greetings in a letter from Philippe Krynen in Bukoba. Since his brave and outspoken attack on the African AIDS orthodoxy there had been moves to remove him from Tanzania. He had appealed to the President. 'The AIDS establishment has not been able to get rid of me,' he wrote.

Now they are trying to get rid of the programme [the Partage project] itself. Why not throw the baby away with the bath water? But it's not so easy. Disgusting letters sent from Tanzania and Brussels [Krynen's charity Partage had received funds from the European Community] are cutting us off from many sponsors. . . . But finance is not all. The local support triggered by all this dirt put on us, has increased tremendously. In the long run we shall be better off when the laboratories are defunded . . . The HIV edifice is seriously cracked as far as I can hear from my bush and [19]95 may see its burial.

A further letter from Bukoba in October 1997 said, 'Due to the failure of the predictions, it [AIDS] is today perceived as a minor health hazard.'

Abidjan, Ivory Coast: US Centers for Disease Control Project

Our last location was Abidjan, Ivory Coast. We knew that Abidjan had become one of the routes from Nigeria for drug smuggling. Because prostitutes are usually in the front line of drug taking, we wanted to find out what effect this might be having on their state of health. We discovered that they were consuming hard drugs in a smokeable form – namely heroin and cocaine, in dangerously adulterated versions. This was a new phenomenon for Africa. These drugs had begun to make their way into Abidjan in 1985/6. They were epidemic among certain classes of prostitutes and these were the ones who were getting ill. Prostitutes addicted to these substances looked as though they had AIDS because they lost a great deal of weight and began to look wasted both from the direct effects of the drugs and because they used what little money they had on drugs rather than food.[38]

The US Centers for Disease Control had based a major research project in Abidjan, headed by Dr Kevin de Cock. Working with him, Dr Georgette Adjorlolo had been running a five-year research project at a maternity clinic in Koumassi. Although more women in Africa are said to be HIV positive (50 per cent of the total whereas in the West 90 per cent are men) what the women do not seem to be showing is a frequent progression to AIDS.

The Koumassi HIV clinic was buzzing with activity the morning we arrived. Gorgeous plump babies were being unwrapped from their back slings by beautiful healthy looking women dressed in vibrant printed cloth. It was hard to believe that all the women there were HIV positive. We were told that 80 per cent of the HIV positive mothers at this clinic were perfectly well. We met and interviewed two mothers and Dr Severin Sibailly commented, 'Generally speaking the two women we have just seen this morning are asymptomatic. They have no signs of AIDS, but the problem is, we don't know when they were infected. But what puzzles us is the fact that many of the women who are classed as negative fulfil the definitions for AIDS.'[39]

Dr Adjorlolo did not doubt that HIV was the cause of AIDS, but she too was puzzled by the differences in progression to AIDS. 'These observations lead me to think that it's not only HIV – but certain co-factors that accelerate the onset of the disease – and maybe other factors such as nutrition and concurrent infections.'[40] Professor Kassi Manlan, a senior health official, had come to a broadly similar conclusion: 'The virus is only a co-factor. One can perhaps say that progression to AIDS is not inevitable – that many people may encounter the human immunodeficiency virus – some will get AIDS, others not.'[41]

All this is a far cry from the messages pushed by international agencies about HIV and AIDS, which millions of Africans had been receiving over the preceding years. The messages on radio accompanied by the roll of the death drums – HIV will get you, AIDS will kill you – struck terror into every listener's heart.

AIDS Without HIV

Of all the accumulating puzzles, the greatest was the increasing number of AIDS cases, defined on clinical grounds, without HIV, *actually documented in science journals*. In September 1992, Duesberg's letter in *Science* drew attention to more than 800 documented US and European clinically diagnosed HIV-free AIDS cases, and upwards of 2200 in Africa that all met the WHO definition of AIDS. There may be more, said Duesberg, and pointed out that only about 50 per cent of all AIDS cases reported by the Centers for Disease Control (CDCs) had been tested for HIV, with diagnoses based on their disease symptoms alone. Of those who *were* tested, 5 per cent never showed signs of HIV.[42]

Furthermore, AIDS researcher Michelle Cochrane, working from Berkeley, had discovered that there could be many, many more HIV-free AIDS cases. She found out that if a person in San Francisco had symptoms of AIDS but the test was negative, he or she would not be entered into the official statistics unless they returned for confirmation of their HIV negative status, which, of course, rarely happened because the majority of those cases never returned and became lost to statistics.[43] Thus, two African studies demonstrating AIDS without HIV are relevant here. In Ghana, of 227 patients suffering weight loss, diarrhoea, chronic fever, tuberculosis and neurological diseases, after antibody tests and supplementary polymerase chain reaction (PCR) tests, 135 (59 per cent) were found to be HIV negative.[44] In Kevin de Cock's studies in three Abidjan hospitals, over one-third of cases *not* qualifying as AIDS under the Bangui definition of symptoms were HIV positive, and one-third of cases that did qualify as AIDS were HIV negative.[45]

When we met Kari Brattegaard, in charge of Kevin de Cock's laboratory, she told us she had performed the usual HIV antibody test (ELISA) on a number of patients with sleeping sickness and had got a 70 per cent HIV positive result. But when she tried to confirm the tests with a second ELISA antibody test she found all the tests were negative. More grist to the mill for our eventual meeting with de Cock himself. My interview with Dr de Cock was somewhat adversarial, to say the least. I asked him how he could explain the 2400 documented cases of AIDS in his and other studies that turned out to be HIV negative? 'If we're talking about AIDS we should perhaps scrap the word and talk about HIV disease. All right. It's very clear what is HIV disease. Now it's not surprising that the constellation of symptoms, signs, and indeed opportunistic infections, occasionally – occasionally – occur in people without HIV infection.' Dr de Cock maintained that those HIV negative cases may have looked like AIDS but they were simply conditions that were drawn into the net when collecting numbers of patients for research purposes (surveillance data) not for patient care. The relevant portion of our interview is worth recording.

Q: *Those 2400 cases were called* AIDS, *for all intents and purposes, in all the literature. And yet you're saying they shouldn't have been called* AIDS. *But they were identical to* AIDS. *So are you saying . . .*

A: *(Dr de Cock) But they were* HIV *negative.*

Q: *So are you saying there have been 2400 misdiagnoses?*

A: *Are you talking about – we're talking about the quality of surveillance data.*

Q: *The documented cases of full-blown* AIDS *which, when tested, were* HIV *negative.*

A: *Well then they're not* AIDS *cases. They're not* AIDS *in the way we talk about* HIV *disease.*

Q: *But they were called* AIDS *in the documents. They were called clinical case definition Bangui* AIDS. *Do you see?*

A: *Of course I see. Any case definition, particularly one which is clinically based is not going to be perfect.*[46]

Bialy's comment on this exchange was: 'When one has clinically identical pictures, one with HIV antibodies, one without HIV antibodies – to call one AIDS and one not AIDS is [a] patent absurdity. This is irrefutable proof that HIV is not necessary for the presence of AIDS, except by definition.'[47] The WHO chose to phrase things differently. When the number of HIV-free AIDS cases became an issue at the Amsterdam world AIDS conference in 1992, and journalists latched on to the fact that the CDC and the NIH had glossed over these figures, the WHO's Global AIDS Programme called a top level meeting in Geneva to discuss the matter. The meeting was chaired by Dr Kevin de Cock. It was announced that cases of HIV-free AIDS were caused by a genetic problem that could lead to irreversible immunodeficiency. They gave this newly concocted disease a name, idiopathic CD4 lymphocytopaenia (ICL). Idiopathic means 'no known cause', so in effect this newly labelled condition simply described the fact that CD4 cells were being killed off for no known reason thus causing immune deficiency.

Anthony Fauci, who was then head of AIDS research at the US NIH, gave his reason for confirming that ICL (or HIV-free AIDS cases) was different from AIDS with HIV. This was that ICL was heterogeneous and affected far more women than those with a similar condition plus HIV (described as AIDS).[48] Duesberg quickly dispelled Fauci's theory in the journal *Bio/Technology* by reminding us that HIV is accepted by the orthodoxy as being the cause of more than 25 heterogeneous diseases and on the point about women, he drew our attention to the fact that the orthodoxy also accepts that HIV causes African AIDS where 50 per cent of the alleged HIV positive cases are women. Thus, there is no difference between ICL (HIV-free AIDS) and what is called AIDS.[49]

The uncertainty behind the science surrounding AIDS in Africa has never been properly exposed. Africans have been hammered over the head for more than a decade with one dreadful certainty, that HIV will kill them. The effect has been like the witch doctor pointing the bone – thousands upon thousands of people have died unnecessarily – psychologically traumatized, stigmatized and neglected. The last word from Africa goes to Dr Martin Okot-Nwang: 'What keeps a man energetic and keeps him doing what he does is his hope for the future. But once you tell me that I am HIV positive then you have given me the message that I am going to die, and therefore I have no energy for the future.'[50]

By the end of 1995, the *Sunday Times* had published an article by Steve Connor, one our most vituperative critics, entitled 'Global drop in aids predicted'. Connor reported:

Scientists are re-examining their predictions about the Aids epidemic after discovering that the explosive spread of the virus has declined in Uganda, one of the world's worst affected countries. [Moreover,] the dramatic fall in the numbers of young people being infected in Uganda follows declining rates in Britain and Thailand, leading to hopes that a worldwide epidemic can be reversed.[51]

Chapter 11

'Diary of an AIDS Dissident'

Battles in Berlin: Berlin World AIDS Conference

I think the truth can be suspended, rerouted, rejected for seemingly astonishingly long periods of time but I think it's like a kind of energy. I don't think it can be destroyed. It is rather like an aeroplane in a holding pattern. It does have to land somewhere, eventually.

(Celia Farber)[1]

I can remember lying flat on my back on the cool stone tiles of Hector's cousin's porch. It was after midnight in a quiet suburb of Berlin. Hector was smoking a cigarette, leaning against the balustrade. We were recovering from the waves of hostility and hatred our presence was creating at the 1993 Berlin World AIDS Conference. It was almost two years since Dr Hector Gildemeister had joined forces with us. He had spent some time as a child in Berlin before settling in England, and eventually graduated from Oxford University with a doctorate in biochemistry. Just as Michael had 'moved in', so had Hector, lending us the support of his considerable intellect and perpetual sense of indignation at the inadequacies of the virus/AIDS hypothesis and its followers. Ever since 1987, world AIDS conferences had come and gone and we had simply read about them in the newspapers. This time, we decided to be there, to observe and to film it. Thus another film, *Diary of an AIDS Dissident* was born, almost on a wing and a prayer, since this time we had applied for network funding.

The two key reasons for our presence in Berlin were to represent the views of several leading scientists deliberately not invited to the conference, who questioned HIV as the cause of AIDS and also to point out that AZT, currently being given to HIV positive people, whether they were ill or not, was highly toxic and had been shown in recent studies to be of no benefit. We had by now made the transition from simple arms-length observers of a scientific discourse to advocates of one side.

The transition did not necessarily sit easily for medical journalists who, like any other journalists, prefer to report on disputes rather than to enter into the fray themselves. But in our case, the virulence of the opposition to our questioning of perceived wisdom was so stark that, in defending our integrity, we had been driven to dig deeper and deeper into the facts and issues supporting our antagonists. And the further we dug the louder the questions that cried out to be asked. Additionally, it has to be said, we found quite distasteful, not to say alarming, the speed and ease with which scientists, whose whole ethos should have depended on curiosity and questioning, could close their minds to the questioning of a hypothesis that at best had so far led nowhere.

As we approached Berlin I realized that we were going to face 14,000 delegates who believed HIV caused AIDS, and hundreds of pharmaceutical company reps with enormous financial interests vested in the virus/AIDS hypothesis. It felt like David and Goliath. On our first evening we met up with the Berlin group of dissidents who had gathered at a pavement cafe with the leading dissident of them all, Peter Duesberg. Ironically, he was in Berlin to visit his mother. Not surprisingly, he had not been invited to the conference and flew back to Berkeley the following day.

We had with us a selection of impressive information dossiers, which included copies of *Rethinking AIDS* with contributions from leading scientists, including Nobel prize winner Kary Mullis, challenging the virus/AIDS hypothesis. We also had Duesberg's latest published paper with its 523 references.[2] We were told we could not display these in the press lounge and the conference organizers quickly confiscated them. This was the beginning of a series of events demonstrating the current of censorship that permeated the conference and stifled any attempt to open a debate that might question HIV as the cause of AIDS and threaten the establishment.

At the opening press conference the chairman, Professor Otto Habermehl, made an important statement, the significance of which may have escaped most of those present. The orthodoxy had so far steadfastly maintained that if you had HIV you would get AIDS and die. But for the first time in such an open forum, Habermehl said not everyone who had HIV would progress to AIDS. The 8 June was one of the hottest days of the year in Berlin. Outside the conference centre stood Christian Joswig, one of the Berlin dissidents, like a brave sentinel, holding up a banner protesting against Wellcome and AZT. Inside the vast air-conditioned complex, Robert Gallo was making his big speech, to be followed by a press conference.

This was the day we were to confront Robert Gallo. We listened to his speech in the press lounge where journalists, eager to take away a little nugget of hope in the battle to target the allegedly mutating virus, watched the TV monitors with an air of bemused stupefaction at Gallo's potpourri of virological mystification-speak stirred in with giant dollops of wishful thinking. 'For the future, it's an exciting theoretical possibility. ... In future this could have dramatic effects. ... You can imagine, theoretically, if that would work, what a great step forward that would be.' There was nothing to hold on to, nothing to write home about and certainly nothing to fill a newspaper column. It was like trying to eat soup with a fork.

The press conference was equally tame – a lot of mutual back-slapping. Then I took my chance. I stood up and quoted Root-Bernstein's point that by the end of the century we would know everything there was to know about HIV but nothing about AIDS. I mentioned Duesberg's contention that none of the predictions based on the HIV hypothesis had come true, and that there had been no heterosexual spread of AIDS. Was it not time to find funding for a total reappraisal of the virus/AIDS hypothesis, not dictated to by the endless search for new, useless and damaging antiviral drugs? Many of my journalist colleagues were heard to hiss with overt disapproval. Gallo paused for a moment. Then he tore at his hair in mock exasperation and replied angrily, 'I think Dr Robert Root-Bernstein doesn't know what he's talking about.' 'I demand a proper answer,' I shouted, as loudly as I could, because they had switched my microphone off. Gallo signalled to the session chairman, press officer Justin Westhoff, that he would comment further:

The answer is, I think he [Root-Bernstein] is wrong. And I think any rational person who is looking at this carefully and slowly has come to the same conclusion – that he is wrong. I don't influence funding. I am not the director of the Institute. I do my work. I work on HIV and the cause of this disease. I have since 1984. If you and Dr Bernstein do not believe it, so be it. Do your work on what you think the cause is and don't bother me.[3]

Many of us knew that Dr Gallo had been under investigation for three years by the US Federal Office of Research Integrity and that in December 1992 he had been found guilty by his peers, of scientific misconduct, a charge he was, at that time, appealing against. It was our Dutch colleague, Robert Laarhoven's turn to ask a question. 'Could you tell me,' he said, 'whether Dr Gallo was accepted as a key speaker at this conference before or after he was found guilty of misconduct, and if after, do you think it is acceptable to have a scientist who has lost credibility addressing us at this moment?' There was more hissing from the audience, at which point Justin Westhoff intervened. 'I am not going to answer it. We will not discuss [it],' he said. 'We should wait for the conference chairman to answer this question.' At the very end, Robert got the following answer, 'Why shouldn't the international conference on AIDS invite two very fruitful AIDS researchers like Professor Montagnier and Dr Gallo?'[4]

The session had a lively ending. Martin Delaney, head of Project Inform in San Francisco and a long-time foe of Duesberg's, became enraged at my questioning the heterosexual spread of AIDS and grabbed my wrist violently. Hector waded in to defend me, quoting the almost non-existent figures for heterosexual spread in the UK. 'I don't care about the UK figures,' Delaney shouted. To which Hector called him a 'silly twit'. Meanwhile, Gallo stormed off the stage, walked straight up to Robert Laarhoven and accused him of being 'cruel' to him. But within seconds he was outside in the main concourse meeting the press photographers. As his bodyguards brutishly shoved journalists aside, Gallo thanked them for protecting him and then switched on his smile for the press.

The Gallo Investigation: Three Separate Inquiries

The Gallo investigation is probably the best example of the way in which a dominant orthodoxy protects its own. Scientific integrity and a genuine desire to discover the truth had little to do with the final outcome of this sorry episode in the history of science. After all, why would the NIH want to see its brightest star in disgrace? Every effort was made to protect Gallo, and this filtered through into the national and scientific press.

How could a scientist who had already been seen to make so many mistakes retain so much power? And how could a flawed hypothesis such as the virus/AIDS one continue to retain so much credibility when so many highly respected scientists have raised so many doubts about it? Why, at the very least, are funding sources not available to doubters? In a truly empirical environment is it not good scientific practice for all reasonable hypotheses to be put to the test? The fact that both Gallo and his hypothesis about AIDS continue to endure is symptomatic of the way in which the process of genuine scientific inquiry has, in itself, become unscientific in Western society.

Over the past decade, power, ambition, greed and vainglory have won the day in the labyrinthine politics and Byzantine intrigue that surround the 'high science' of molecular biology. The most powerful man of the decade has been Robert Gallo himself. Described by *Newsweek* as one of America's 25 'leading innovators', Gallo has won more than 80 prizes in his career and has presided over a laboratory of some 50 scientists with a budget of $13 million. But although his laboratory has been described by a government official as 'the cutting edge of science', looking through more than 100 relevant articles in our archive, it is clear that he was unpopular with most of his former colleagues.

Fierce rivalries and jealousies will always abound in the hothouse world of highly financed science laboratories. The stories about Gallo's laboratory are legion and the recurring theme is one of disappointment among his assistants about due recognition and attribution surrounding their work. To find what became identified as HIV, a permanent (or immortalized) cell line was required in which HIV could replicate. This procedure had to be carried out in the laboratory. It had proved notoriously difficult in the past to produce the right permanent cell line.

In a hard-hitting article in *Science* by Ellis Rubinstein, we read how the scientists who originally cultured the permanent cell line Gallo used to find HIV felt about their treatment. When HIV is being looked for in blood taken from a patient it can only be found after being cultured in the laboratory using a permanent cell line. These cell lines are usually cancer cells. They are taken from individual patients and kept going in the laboratory. They are often named after the patient's initials. Scientists Adi Gazdar, Paul Bunn, John Minna, Bernard Poiesz and Frank Ruscetti all contributed to the growth of a permanent cell line called HUT78 in which HIV could replicate.

This was the cell line that was used in Gallo's laboratory by his chief virologist Mikulas Popovic to find HIV. However, in the Gallo laboratory HUT78 mysteriously changed its name to H9, thus allowing it to be distanced from those who had originally cultured it. Gallo's AIDS papers published in *Science* claimed that H9 was a derivative of a new cell line called HT. But John Crewdson's search through laboratory documents, released through the freedom of information procedure, confirmed that Popovic's handwritten laboratory notes showed that he had changed the name HUT78 to HT in December 1983.[5]

Gazdar made a formal complaint to the NIH. He appealed for recognition of the use of his own cell line and consideration of his right to income from the Gallo NIH patent. 'It's not only money,' he told *Science*, 'it's attribution. Here's a line that is used worldwide for AIDS testing and no one knows that it came from my laboratory.' Writes Rubinstein, 'But Gallo told *Science* that Gazdar's plea for credit is a 'pathetic joke'. Says Gallo: 'I don't consider it so brilliant. In my mind there is no credit for a cell line. If it happens by accident that you have a cell line, so freaking what? We didn't patent a cell line; we patented the process.' Later in the article Gallo is quoted as saying:

I've got to be worrying and focusing on whether we could have definitely proven in 1985 instead of 1987 that this [HIV] was derived from HUT78? Maybe so – God knows we were saying that it was probable. The fact is we could have. . . . The fact is I never really thought it was important. And quite frankly I still don't and I don't understand the people who do.[6]

Well, Gazdar may have thought that two years' worth of patent revenue at $100,000 a year was important.

Gallo Under Fire

The initial dispute between Montagnier and Gallo as to who first discovered HIV was settled in 1987 when French and US lawyers hammered out a compromise agreement whereby the $8 million earned annually from royalties for the HIV blood test patent would be shared. But the situation rumbled on for another two years until, like a clap of thunder, investigative journalist John Crewdson unleashed his 50,000-word attack on Gallo in the *Chicago Tribune*. He described Gallo as 'an influential and intimidating scientist who chased the wrong virus for more than a year, only to reverse course and emerge with a virtual genetic twin of the virus that had already been discovered by his rivals in Paris and delivered to him months before.' Crewdson concluded that Gallo obtained the AIDS virus from Montagnier's laboratory either by 'accident or theft'.[7]

This led to calls from the Pasteur Institute (Montagnier's laboratory) to renegotiate the 1987 agreement and to ask for $20 million in reparation. It also led Congressman John Dingell, a much feared whistleblower in the corridors of science, to demand an immediate investigation. Dingell had already been investigating scientific and financial misconduct by members of Gallo's team. Now, in a letter to Gallo's boss, acting director of the NIH, William Raub, Dingell roared, 'in the past NIH has turned a blind eye to misconduct by senior scientists supported by Federal funds. We trust this will not be the case in the present situation, and that the allegations will be thoroughly investigated and appropriate actions taken if warranted.'[8]

Raub replied that an inquiry was underway by the NIH's Office of

Scientific Integrity of their own star researcher, Robert Gallo. A panel of 11 scientists appointed by the National Academy of Scientists was in charge of it. By October 1990 the inquiry was converted into a formal investigation and it was also to include Gallo's chief virologist, Mikulas Popovic, who had been responsible for growing viruses in Gallo's laboratory during the critical 1983/4 period.

There were at least 12 points under investigation, including charges of missing data, unwillingness to credit other scientists' contributions and false denials that HIV had been used in Popovic's virus cultures. Mikulas Popovic had adopted unusual methods to culture HIV. He had pooled ten viruses from ten patients and then cultured them. One damning piece of evidence had already emerged through John Crewdson's investigations. James Swire, lawyer for the Pasteur Institute, had received a letter written to Popovic by an electromicroscopist at the National Cancer Institute who had been studying cells containing viruses from Gallo's laboratory. The original version of the letter, dated 14 December 1983, said that the French virus LAV had been successfully photographed growing in cultures. But when Swire received a further copy of that letter in response to a freedom of information request in 1985, all mention of LAV had been deleted. Gallo later denied any knowledge of this.

The situation was further complicated by Gallo's claim that both Montagnier's and Gallo's HIV samples had become contaminated with blood from another patient called Lai. So what, said Gallo, in a letter to *Nature* echoing with moral self-righteousness. The similarity between his virus and Montagnier's 'now seems to be explained ... in short none of this affects the history of the important events written for *Nature* in 1987 and *Scientific American* in 1988 by Luc Montagnier and myself. It is now time for this period of controversy to come to an end and for us all to focus our efforts on ending the pandemic.'[9]

But the matter could not so easily be brushed aside. Simon Wain-Hobson, a researcher at the Pasteur Institute said, 'We all knew it was a contamination back in 1986. Why did it take him [Gallo] six years to admit it? We made a blood test from a virus isolated in France, Gallo made a blood test from the same virus isolated in France. These are the facts.'[10] Meanwhile, Representative John Dingell was still on the warpath. Frustrated by the failure so far to obtain a conclusion of scientific misconduct, Dingell shifted the focus of his attack on Gallo from misconduct to perjury and patent fraud, in association with Gallo's application for his HIV test patent.

On 31 December 1992 the *New York Times* published a front page report announcing the results of the Office of Research Integrity's inquiry. Both Gallo and Popovic were found guilty of scientific misconduct. The investigators said Gallo had 'falsely reported' a critical fact in his scientific paper of 1984, and had intentionally misled colleagues to gain credit for himself and diminish credit due to his French competitors. The report also said that his false statement had 'impeded potential AIDS research progress' by diverting scientists from potentially fruitful work with the French researchers.[11]

Gallo and his lawyers had been able to set aside most of the original points of inquiry, whittling them down to the three on which he was found guilty, which concentrated on Gallo's 1984 paper announcing his discovery of HIV. Popovic denied any culpability. Gallo's comment through his lawyer, Joe Onek, was that despite a long and intensive investigation, 'ORI could only take issue with a few trivial mistakes and a single sentence written by me.' The finding that the sentence is false, said Gallo, 'is utterly unwarranted. It is based on a distorted interpretation of the sentence.' Gallo said the investigation findings 'have no bearing on the validity and importance of the research on AIDS conducted by my laboratory'.[12] Both Gallo and Popovic decided to appeal against the findings.

This was the stage things were at when Robert Laarhoven raised the question of Gallo's presence at the Berlin World AIDS Conference. But by the time we had finished editing our film, in November 1993, the situation had changed again. The Department of Health and Human Services appeals board (made up of lawyers, not scientists) looked into Popovic's case first and decided on new criteria for the definition of scientific misconduct. 'Intent to deceive' had to be proved. On this basis the ORI decided it had to drop Gallo's case and charges of misconduct were withdrawn. The goal posts had been moved yet again to protect the orthodoxy.

I can remember telephoning a disconsolate Lyle Bivens, head of the

NIH's Office of Research Integrity. When I asked him how he felt about withdrawing the charges of misconduct against Gallo he said, 'I do not consider this a victory. We do not agree with the standards applied by the appeals board, which are working to protect the interests of scientists.' He told me that there was no doubt that Gallo had been found guilty of misconduct by his scientific peers and that the ORI still maintained the facts of the case. 'He [Gallo] has acknowledged that he was in error ... Between you and me, unless you come to the wrong conclusion in your study, you can get away with anything.'

Results of the Concorde Trial: AZT Shows No Benefit in Asymptomatics

After the Gallo session ended, I bumped into a familiar face on the concourse. It was Professor Kassi Manlan, whom we had met in the Ivory Coast. He beamed when he saw us and then his face clouded. 'I am shocked by what I see here. African people are being humiliated at this conference'. He had attended several sessions dealing with AIDS prevention in Africa. 'All I could see was white women rolling condoms on to big black penises. It is *très dégoûtant*. It seems to me that AIDS has given people free reign to talk about sex in public. And that is all they do. The atmosphere is both salacious and degrading.'

One of the most important issues at the conference was AZT and the publication of the results of the Concorde study. In April, two months before the conference, the results of the three-year Concorde study had been published in the *Lancet*. Concorde had tried to find out if there was any benefit in giving AZT early to HIV positive individuals who had no symptoms of AIDS, rather than later on when symptoms began to emerge. The group that received AZT early was called the 'immediate group' and that given the drug later the 'deferred group'. The trial, conducted jointly in Paris and London, involving 1749 participants, concluded, 'Concorde has not shown any significant benefit from the immediate use of zidovudine [AZT] compared with deferred therapy in symptom-free individuals in terms of survival or disease progression.'[13]

This was a severe blow to Wellcome, which had been pushing the early use of AZT for several years, and a severe blow to all recently diagnosed HIV positives who may have believed that AZT would help them. Not only did AZT not help, according to Concorde, but it caused *more* serious side effects and there were *more* deaths in the group that had been subjected to AZT longest. To be precise, 95 people died in the early (immediate) group and 76 in the late (deferred) group – the group not given AZT until the patients had begun to develop symptoms. A further blow came when the MRC issued its press release about Concorde. The MRC, which had conducted the trial together with its French counterpart INSERM, announced that although four previous similar studies, three of which were terminated early after less than a year, had found a delay in the clinical progression to AIDS, 'such a delay was not seen [in Concorde] over the longer follow-up period.'[14]

Concern about the possible toxic effects of AZT on babies and small children had led to demonstrations a few weeks earlier outside Great Ormond Street Hospital for Sick Children. This was the centre of a trial headed by Professor Catherine Peckham and Dr Diana Gibb, called Paediatric European Network for Treatment in AIDS – PENTA I Trial,[15] which planned to give AZT to more than 300 HIV positive babies across Europe with no symptoms of AIDS. Many of the babies already recruited into the trial in the UK were born to African mothers with limited grasp of English. Some of the women had become very worried about their children being given AZT, for they had heard about its toxic effects.

I was asked to report on this issue for Sky News[16] and met several of the African mothers whose children were in the trial. Two had decided to withdraw from the trial and had thrown away the AZT syrup for their children. Another two told me that they were afraid AZT would damage their children but did not dare pull out. George Galloway MP had taken up the issue and told me, 'If people knew that this highly toxic drug was being administered to potentially hundreds of small children – as I say, most of them black, most of them without a voice, their parents without a voice in British society, then I think these tests would be stopped and I think the whole situation ought to be investigated by the Government.'[17]

At one of the Berlin press conferences, Niki Adams from the English

Collective of Prostitutes, brought the issue up with Ian Weller, 'In the light of the Concorde study, do you not consider that there should be a thorough reevaluation of the PENTA study? ... Would you go as far as saying that the trials should be stopped immediately?' Weller replied, 'I would think people would be wrong to extrapolate the results in an adult trial to the child model. ... Therefore I would support the continuation of trials in children of that age group.' 'Even when they are asymptomatic?' asked Niki. Weller, who had earlier said he himself would not give AZT to asymptomatic adult patients replied, 'Even when they are asymptomatic, yes.'[18]

It was at this moment that the news began to spread that there had been an incident outside involving the gay activist group Act Up. Act Up members were in Berlin as 'official dissidents'. We had been told that week that Act Up in the UK had received £60,000 from Wellcome, which many members had used to pay for their trip to Berlin. The UK contingent took umbrage at Christian Joswig's anti-Wellcome, anti-AZT posters, snatched them from him and burned them.

Peter Schmidt, Joswig's colleague who had been filming the goings on for his AIDS dissident programme on Berlin's access cable channel, was ordered to erase the footage from his tape by the German police. Meanwhile, the police had ordered Robert Laarhoven to leave the stand he was manning in the conference hall and had taken him outside. If he attempted to re-enter the conference hall he would be arrested. A furious Laarhoven said, 'It became clear to me there is very heavy censorship of dissident information and I am not afraid any more to use words like "AIDS fascism".'[19] The tension of the last few days had begun to take its toll. No longer did any of us smile. The hostility was so powerful, even among our own journalist fraternity, that all we could do every morning was set our faces into a concrete mould and wade through the sea of scowling faces.

We had been joined by Celia Farber the journalist who had taken up the cause of AIDS. 'When I walk around here I feel like this is so hopeless,' she said. 'What we are up against is a gargantuan multimillion dollar infrastucture. Who do we think we are? Whom do we think we are kidding? We have to be like Sysiphus rolling the ball up the hill and let it roll down the other side.'[20] So we rolled the ball up the hill to the last press conference.

Would Professor Habermehl (the conference chairman) apologize for the horrible acts of violence and censorship at the conference, asked Lauritsen? Habermehl gave him a straight 'No'. At the opening press briefing Habermehl had described people who questioned the role of HIV as 'mentally unstable'. It was Celia's turn to take up the cudgels. She reminded Habermehl that there were many distinguished scientists in the Group for the Scientific Reappraisal of HIV. 'You refer to Dr Mullis [Nobel prize winner and inventor of polymerase chain reaction],' said Celia, 'who is one of your colleagues as "mentally unstable". If you were not aware of this, now that you have been made aware of it, would you consider an apology?' 'I would like to give you a statement,' said Habermehl. 'I think it was not a good way to say "mentally disturbed" and I will change it. I will say "bizarre".'[21]

London: AZT on Trial Conference

We had formed a group in London in early 1993 called SCAM (Standing Committee on AZT Malpractice) chaired by writer Martin Walker, author of *Dirty Medicine*.[22] The aim of the group was to organize a London conference on AZT that would highlight the issues surrounding Concorde and the PENTA trial. The London gay press had not been cooperative and the Pink Paper had actually withdrawn our advertisement for the conference.

On the morning of 20 June 1993, at Kingsway College in London, Martin Walker opened the proceedings with a speech about the way multinationals like Wellcome can use their influence:

What we are talking about is the product marketing of a very expensive overcapitalized product which has got to be sold on and has got to make something in the region of £400 million or £600 million in the first three or four years of its existence. It normally takes a period of anything between five to twelve years for a new drug to obtain a license. AZT was fast-tracked though the British licensing system even though there had been no trials in Britain.[23]

There were many young men present who had been personally involved in the AIDS and AZT debate. Pascal de Bock, who had been a volunteer in our office for a year, told us he had to give up his job as an operating theatre charge nurse when he was diagnosed HIV positive. He took AZT for three years and then suffered a stroke.

I said, well, if AZT had been given to me for three years and had not done anything for my T4 cell count or for my health, there is something wrong there. I decided therefore to bin every single medication I was on. So I just binned the migraine medication, the HIV medication, everything. I learned from another group [Positively Healthy] how to regain my responsibility for my health and therefore I have been more alive.[24]

Four years on Pascal is in good health.

It was at this conference that Duesberg, who had arrived from San Francisco, focused on important new information. He targeted the statutory information produced by Wellcome for the UK Data Sheet Compendium and the American Physicians' Desk Reference (PDR). It was wrong, he announced. Earlier studies by Robert Gallo and Sam Broder claimed that AZT could target HIV and was 1000 times more toxic to HIV than it was to healthy human cells. These findings had led to recommended dosage levels in doctors' manuals. 'But in the meantime,' said Duesberg, 'a number of investigators have also checked the toxicity of AZT and found that Dr Gallo had made an error by a factor of 1000. This is not a minor little error.'[25] In other words, AZT was 1000 times more toxic to healthy cells than had hitherto been claimed.

'So,' continued Duesberg, 'Gallo faithfully believed and so did Burroughs Wellcome and Broder, that AZT therapy was justified because AZT is 1000 times less toxic to the cell than it is to the virus. So that belief clearly must be questioned now because that result could not be reproduced by four independent studies.'[26] Duesberg's assertions were then reported to the MRC in connection with SCAM's complaints about the PENTA studies. No action was forthcoming.

Although the AZT on Trial conference attracted more than 200 delegates from all over the world, it made little impact on the national and gay press. But, a few weeks after the conference there came support from an unexpected source. *Capital Gay* carried an article written by its ex-editor, and at that moment acting editor, Graham McKerrow – its title, 'It's time to lift the censorship'. 'I write as the editor who invented AIDS journalism in this country,' he said lamenting the current dearth of 'shades of opinion' in the reporting of AIDS in the gay press, which relied too much on so-called AIDS experts. He said it was now time 'our press habitually referred to HIV as "the *suspected* cause of AIDS" [emphasis added].'[27]

AZT and Babies: The PENTA Trial

The focus of our filming now turned to the administration of AZT to HIV positive pregnant mothers, babies and children. A study in the USA (ACTG 076) giving AZT to pregnant mothers had been abandoned. It involved the administration of intravenous AZT to mothers in labour, and babies at birth were given AZT syrup. Under pressure from Neenya Ostrum of the *New York Native*, the trialists revealed data from the first 30 women. This showed that 10 per cent of the children born to these women had rare birth defects. Some were born with extra fingers and toes. And five babies were born with neutropaenia, a decrease in a type of white blood cell (a known AZT side effect) which apparently reversed itself.[28]

We continued with our investigation into the PENTA trial in London and elsewhere in Europe where AZT was being given to HIV positive babies with no symptoms of AIDS, even though the Concorde trial had showed no benefit for adults in the same circumstances. We learned that out of 35 children given AZT in the PENTA trial, 15 had developed blood disorders because of a toxic effect on their bone marrow; in seven this was serious enough to require blood transfusions. The purpose of PENTA was to find out when to start giving AZT to babies and children. Dr Richard Nicholson, editor of the *Bulletin of Medical Ethics* said, 'What on earth is the point of continuing with a trial to find the correct time to start AZT in HIV positive children when you haven't conclusive evidence that AZT does the children good at any stage?'[29]

A picket was organized by SCAM – together with GAG (Gays against

Genocide), The English Collective of Prostitutes and Black Women for Wages for Housework – for 15 September 1993 outside the MRC's London headquarters to protest against the trials and a letter calling for an end to the trial was handed in to an MRC representative. That day the MRC issued a press release accusing the demonstrators of causing distress to the families of sick children and of distributing 'scare-mongering leaflets, the contents of which bear little relation to the truth, and personal attacks on doctors who are involved in the trial and whose only concern is to find the best treatment for their patients.'[30]

SCAM continued with its preparation of an extensive document in collaboration with doctors and scientists with detailed objections to PENTA based on a new analysis of AZT's toxicity.[31] There were many problems with the PENTA trial's protocol[32] that worried the experts we had consulted (see Appendix B). One of the key concerns was that if a child, whether on a placebo or on the drug failed to thrive, and 'definitely needs AZT' it should automatically be put on AZT. Thus, if the child was receiving AZT already, it would be continued, and if it was on the dummy (placebo) it would be put on AZT therapy. (This is called open label transfer.) As the effects of AZT are often indistin-guishable from the symptoms of AIDS itself, it would not be possible to know whether a child was genuinely failing to thrive, or suffering from the effects of AZT. If the latter, it could be very dangerous to keep it on the drug.

A delegation from SCAM delivered the dossier to the MRC head-quarters on 1 December 1993 together with a letter from George Galloway: 'I wish to say that I have grave worries about these [PENTA] trials which are, of course, being part funded by yourselves along with money from the European Community. ... The MRC with its huge importance in British public life and its Hippocratical concern for medical ethics should halt these trials forthwith.'[33]

In February 1994 came the MRC's response: it would not be address-ing the issue of toxicity. The reason given was by now very familiar to us all: 'AZT has been licensed for use in symptomatic disease by the regulatory authorities in the UK, USA and many other countries, follow-ing detailed study of the toxicity data; they also keep studies under review in the light of subsequent information. It would therefore be inappropriate for the Council to comment on the general toxicity data.'[34] The PENTA trial is still ongoing as I write.

When transmission of *Diary of an AIDS Dissident* on Sky News finally came in December 1993, the results were predictable. A live phone in after the programme, skilfully handled by Laurie Meyer revealed a tirade of indignant callers accusing us of heresy. But Chris Dunkley's response to the programme in the *Financial Times* showed that at least some headway was being made in getting our message across. Making a comparison with Copernicus under the Roman Catholic Church and dissidents in Russia, which ought to have made us blush with modesty had we not become so enraged by the machinations of the AIDS orthodoxy, Dunkley described the attempts to question the conventional wisdom on AIDS as:

an uphill move against entrenched dogma, amour propre *and, most resistant of all, political correctness. . . . And yet things are beginning to look up. . . . Being told 'Any fool can see the sun goes round the earth and your denial makes you an atheist' or 'any fool can see communism works and your denial makes you a lunatic' must sound to [the programme makers] very much like 'any fool can see* HIV *causes* AIDS, *the pandemic in sub-Saharan Africa proves that homosexuality is not a factor,* AZT *is a useful treatment, and your denial makes you a homophobe.' . . . But the revelation that members of the* AIDS *establishment are now so nervous that they are trying to suppress dissident publications suggests that we may be near to a breakthrough of the truth in the larger public domain.*[35]

But breakthroughs in the AIDS saga curiously are never trumpeted when their effect is to weaken the orthodox hypothesis. So the short report that appeared in the February 1995 issue of the *Lancet* caused hardly a stir. It announced that the US NIH ACTG152 trial giving children AZT and a similar chain terminator drug called ddI had been halted. 'Death rates, growth failure, opportunistic infections and neurological and neurodevelopmental deterioration were commoner in the zidovudine (AZT) group.'[36]

Chapter 12

Whatever Happened to AIDS in Haiti?

T he veranda at the Oloffson Hotel was full on the evening we arrived. The hotel, a graceful wooden great house, built as a family home by the Sam family and still run by its members, provides an indispensable oasis for travellers and, this month, for the world's international correspondents gathered there to await the forthcoming elections, only three weeks away.

There had been rioting in the streets the week before – 12 wounded and 7 dead. Demonstrators wanted President Aristide to run for another three years; the three years of his last elected period were spent in exile in the USA after the military coup. Tensions were high. It was like Graham Greene in high gear. At every table journalists were tapping away at their laptops or murmuring confidentially to their contacts, peering around over hands cupped to the mouth. The fan danced lazily over our heads as the waiters slipped silently between the tables. So there we were, having brazenly driven across the border from the Dominican Republic – James Whitehead, a young gay English researcher on AIDS, Kenny Padilla, our guide from the Dominican Republic and I, doing research into AIDS in Haiti. This, everybody at the Oloffson found very puzzling indeed.

Haiti, one of the poorest countries in the world, had in the early 1980s been expected to infect the rest of the world with AIDS. It was widely reported that its own population would be devastated by this plague. How had Haiti, with a population of 7 million, become blamed for spreading AIDS into the West? And how had Haitians as a nation become categorized as one of the original '4H Club' of haemophiliacs, heroin users, homosexuals and Haitians, who were most at risk of AIDS?

There were many now discredited theories; the most absurd linked AIDS in Haiti with Africa and claimed that African monkeys, possible carriers of AIDS, were imported into Haiti and kept as pets in brothels.[1] Another theory developed in Randy Shilts's book *And the Band Played On*, pointed to a certain 'patient zero', a highly sexually active gay airline steward, Gaetan Dugas, who went to Haiti and allegedly spread AIDS across America and Europe.[2] During the 1970s, Haiti had indeed become the Caribbean playground for American gay men willing to pay young Haitian boys for sex. Many of these tourists were already suffering from sexually transmitted diseases before their Haitian adventures, and later when their immune systems could no longer bear the repeated assaults, became very ill. However, this did not implicate Haiti as a specific AIDS risk.

The story of how a group of very sick Haitians in a Miami hospital became tagged with the AIDS label and led to a whole nation being described as an AIDS risk can be described in a few sentences. It involves principally three men; Michael Gottlieb, a researcher into T-cells in Los Angeles, Wayne Shandera of the Los Angeles EIS and James Curran at the US Centers for Disease Control (CDC), Atlanta, Georgia. In their zeal to enlarge upon an original small cluster of gay men with Kaposi's sarcoma (KS), pneumocystis carinii pneumonia (PCP) and low T-cell counts, calls were made around the USA looking for other similar cases with low T-cell counts.

When Jackson Memorial Hospital in Miami received a call from the CDC asking if they had seen any cases of homosexual men who were severely immune-suppressed, the reply was 'no', but the hospital did describe cases of undernourished Haitian boat people who had arrived with a virulent form of TB, salmonellosis, and a variety of gut parasites leading to diarrhoea and malnutrition. There were also cases of toxoplasmosis, common in Haiti, candida albicans (thrush) and PCP (pneumocystis carinii pneumonia, which before the advent of HIV was normally associated with malnutrition). These Haitian patients were severely immune suppressed and many were not responding to treatment. The cases were quickly added to others from King's County Hospital in New York and from then on, supposedly, the risk of AIDS was no longer limited to homosexual men. Simply to be Haitian meant to be at risk of AIDS and to be unsuitable as a blood donor. Further fuel was added to anti-Haitian prejudice by a subsequent series of post-mortems carried out by the hospital in Miami which showed many women and children with widely disseminated internal Kaposi's sarcoma.

The effect of all this on Haiti was dramatic. The tourist industry collapsed and with it the economy. In the USA, Haitians all over the country lost their jobs. Incensed by this, Haiti's Minister of Health, Ari Bordes, demanded that the Centers for Disease Control strike Haiti off their list of risk categories. The CDC reluctantly agreed and, with a little juggling of statistics, reallocated the Haitians to different specific disease risk groups. But one big misunderstanding took many years to clear up. Those early Haitian patients in the USA, when asked if they were homosexual, denied it vehemently. In Haiti, if a man is asked to pleasure another man, he expects to be paid and does not regard himself as homosexual. In Western terms he would be described as a gay male prostitute, but they don't see it that way.

One of Haiti's leading intellectuals, Dr Joli-coer, regularly to be seen at the Oloffson Hotel in dapper dark suit with silver knobbed cane, had lived through the whole period. 'Haiti has been greatly damaged by AIDS,' he said angrily:

We don't see any epidemic here, but now that all their predictions are wrong, they [the Americans] do nothing to put things right. They got the whole thing wrong. They questioned Haitians in Miami hospitals and those Haitians denied they were homosexual. They did not want to admit they were either homosexual or bisexual.[3] So everyone believed that Haitians got AIDS without being homosexual. But these men were prostitutes and had been in contact with US tourists who were homosexual. The Haitians that got sick were the ones that were in touch with the tourists. These same people were also in contact with the drugs scene, so I think it was the drugs that were 'contagious' and affected their health.

Feeling out of place in the atmosphere of menace and intrigue at the Oloffson Hotel, we were glad to be on our way up the hill behind Port au Prince past some of the few remaining *fin-de-siècle* wooden great houses, past some modern concrete mansions to Manuel Duce's HQ. He worked for Médecins Sans Frontières and his team lived and worked out of an airy house at the top of the hill.

Manuel Duce, a classically handsome Spaniard with a mop of light brown hair, is a nutritionist who with his team from the charity ACSUR Las Segovias, was setting up a series of medicine dispensaries in a rural province in central Haiti, funded by the European Union. There were no medicines available to anyone in the rural areas. The idea was to select suitable candidates to run the dispensaries paid for by the WHO, which supplied a week's training and an initial free supply of essential drugs like antibiotics, TB and anti-parasitic medicines.

In the 11 months he had been working in Haiti, Duce had made a startling observation, 'I hear people talking about AIDS but I have never seen one case of confirmed AIDS,' he told me. Sick people, yes. TB was endemic and there was a marked increase in typhoid fever. Children in his area suffered an average of seven severe diarrhoeas in a year and many suffered from respiratory tract infections (pneumonias accounting for 24 per cent of child mortality) and malnutrition. There was therefore an urgent need for his project's dispensaries, for no proper medication was reaching his people. But as far as Duce was concerned, all the AIDS money pouring into Haiti from the WHO, and America's USAID, earmarked for sex education programmes and condom distribution was completely misdirected. 'People just don't use condoms here,' he said. 'It is a waste of money and a waste of condoms.'

At the beginning of 1993, according to WHO figures, 20,000 HIV positive cases in Haiti had been reported (60 per cent male and 40 per cent female). The HIV seroprevalence in urban areas was estimated at 5–10 per cent and in rural areas at 2–6 per cent. These were the figures that were constantly quoted at us by the AIDS organizations. Yet the actual WHO figures for reported AIDS cases in Haiti over 15 years, from 1979 to 1994 totalled 4967 – and that from a country supposedly the Western epicentre for a deadly epidemic. Here was evidence of the customary juggling with figures by AIDS agencies keen to inflate the numbers by quoting estimates for HIV positive people rather than figures for reported AIDS cases.

When we visited Port au Prince General Hospital to inquire into their AIDS experience, we were surprised to be told that there was no specific AIDS ward at the hospital. 'People come to the hospital very sick with TB, malaria, dysentery,' said a pleasant young doctor 'Some get tested and some are found to be HIV positive,' she shrugged. Exploring the issue of HIV testing in Haiti was obviously going to be a key to our investigation. The National Laboratory Research Institute was where most of the HIV testing in Haiti was undertaken. The laboratories were also the centre for the GHESKIO project. GHESKIO stands for the Haitian Group on Kaposi's Sarcoma and Opportunistic Infections. Funded by, among others, Cornell University, the WHO (which pays for most of the tests), USAID (which pays for most of the sex counselling and family planning) and UNICEF, GHESKIO provided free HIV testing for Haitian people.

Dr Marie Deschamps was one of Haiti's brightest stars in the field. She had worked on the project for 15 years and was obviously a dedicated and diligent researcher. Again, I was reminded how, whenever meeting someone like Dr Deschamps, I would be amazed at the way the religion of HIV and its alleged infectivity made even the most intelligent people incapable of or unwilling to see the AIDS picture from a fresh angle – even when none of the predictions and figures quoted actually stood up to full scrutiny. When the dubious value of the evidence linking HIV with AIDS stared them in the face every effort would always be made to create excuses for anomalies and to find ways of wriggling out of patently untenable situations.

According to Dr Deschamps there were no figures for AIDS in Haiti, only figures for people who were HIV positive ('HIV disease' had become the fashionable phrase). In fact a fundraising letter for the centre's AIDS work was careful only to quote WHO world estimates for HIV positive people (40 million by the year 2000) and an estimated figure of 6500 orphans who, the letter states, would exist in Port au Prince because of AIDS. As so often happens with AIDS researchers, the talk with Deschamps was all in percentages. For example, Deschamps told us that the estimated number of HIV positives (seroprevalence) in

Haiti prior to 1991 had been about 6 per cent and after 1991 had remained stable at 8–9 per cent of a population of 7 million. About 40 per cent of those had been tested. The remaining 60 per cent were based on clinical diagnoses without a test. Her laboratories performed double ELISA HIV tests but no Western blot (the test commonly used in the West to confirm ELISA results). Ironically, Western blot has now been abandoned in the UK as a confirmatory test and a double ELISA on the latest generation test kits is considered to be the most reliable way of testing for HIV.

Of the 2000 blood samples that were sent to her laboratory for testing every month, about half were HIV positive. Dr Deschamps was worried that their very latest testing kits manufactured by Abbott, which were supposed to test for both HIV1 and HIV2, were causing problems. The first test was giving a 'weak reaction' and when repeated with a second they were 'not automatically reactive', meaning they were negative or indeterminate. However, when she performed the second test using the older test kit manufactured by Pasteur laboratories, she obtained a positive result. All of this seemed to confirm – although Dr Deschamps couldn't see it that way – the sham of HIV testing. Without a gold standard (no actually isolated virus) against which to compare each test kit, errors can become compounded instead of evened out. It is quite possible therefore that the vast majority of HIV testing in Third World countries produces false positives, owing both to anomalies in the test kits themselves and also to the fact that people who live in areas where leprosy, malaria, TB and lupus are common, can produce false positive HIV test results.

We asked Dr Deschamps what the latency period was for progressing to full blown AIDS. She said about five to seven years. Did she think everyone would die who was positive? Everyone, she pronounced. The fact that these predictions simply hadn't materialized and that hundreds of thousands of AIDS deaths should have occurred, which had not occurred, did not phase Dr Deschamps. The population in Haiti had been increasing steadily and, as we knew from our African experience, there were no figures for registered deaths with which to compare. The certainty of HIV = AIDS = death was firmly embedded in this scientist.

Dr Deschamps went on to announce that a paper she had prepared would be published in the *Lancet* shortly. It described an eight-year study of 920 sexually-active couples (condoms are not normally used in Haiti, she told us). Of these couples, 475 were 'discordant', that is to say one partner was positive and one negative. 'After eight years,' she said, amazed at her own findings, very few of those couples became 'concordant' that is both partners becoming HIV positive. 'What do you mean by very few?' we asked. 'Only 36 couples,' she replied. That means that over a period of eight years 439 couples did not 'infect' each other. 'I can't really explain it,' she said. The closed mind, rooted in the accepted wisdom on HIV and AIDS, had to look for explanations within her own hypothesis. Where was the scientist's curiosity, we again wondered, that might have yielded explanations other than the accepted wisdom? Where was the inclination at least to listen to those who doubted the infectivity of HIV? What had happened to doubt and questioning among scientists?

There remained only to find some AIDS cases. So we set out for Mother Teresa's hospice, the Missionaries of Charity at St Martin. St Martin is on the hill above the old market. We wound our way through the market in our car and became hopelessly ensnared between enormous vibrantly painted country buses with giant menacing bumpers and a myriad of trucks and small vehicles. There was no road. There was just a sea of people. *Là bas! A droite! A gauche!*, said the people we stopped to ask the way. But how? I asked. Where is the road? Just put your foot down on the accelerator and you will see, they answered. So Kenny did, and like the parting of the Red Sea, wave upon wave of traders gathered up their baskets and wares and made way for us, only to fold back seamlessly together when we had gone through.

We were getting nowhere, until Kenny spotted a little nun in neat grey habit trotting purposefully along, carrying a plastic shopping bag. James jumped out of the car and begged her to help us. Sister Marie Eugénie Beaulice of the Sisters of Mary came to our rescue. She gave up her trip to the Silesian monastery, jumped into our car and led us to the Missionaries of Charity hospice. The mother superior, Sister Sunupa, was from India and wore the familiar white toque edged with dark blue bands. She would be happy to take us round the hospice and told us about her work as we walked to the wards. Here was a woman who in all innocence was doing everything in her power to help destitute members of the community who were very sick. No one could criticize her for the disturbing facts we were about to hear. But the scientists, doctors and politicians who have unquestioningly perpetrated a relentless and unquestioning orthodoxy on AIDS have much to answer for.

Sister Sunupa told us that everyone who came to this shelter had TB, young and old, and many had parasites and other infectious diseases. Because her charity had enough money to test for HIV, everyone was given a blood test. She said 90 per cent turned out to be HIV positive. 'Because we know they will definitely die of AIDS,' she continued, 'we have decided we cannot afford to give our HIV positive patients medication.' There it was. The awful truth in one short sentence. All those people, many of them young, with treatable infections, were being denied medicines that could save their lives. Because the only funding available was for HIV testing, HIV testing became the order of the day. And because immune systems had been damaged by TB, it was not surprising that so many 'tests' proved positive. These people had come here to be helped. But their presence here under the watchful eyes of truly benevolent and well intentioned carers was condemning them to death.

The men's ward was full and there were one or two young men who looked very emaciated and close to death. The rest were ambulant, many of them elderly. It was the women's ward that caused us the greatest anguish. It was full of young, often plump, healthy-looking women, sitting disconsolately on their beds. They had probably been told the results of their HIV test and the death drums were already sounding in their ears. Some of them managed a brief smile. I was allowed to take photographs, and two of them posed for me beside the statue of the Virgin Mary. It was with sadness that we parted. I liked the lively, humorous Sister Sunupa and wished her well in her lonely work among some of the poorest and sickest people in the world. What else could one do?

The second biggest project in Haiti is based at St Catherine's Hospital in a slum suburb of Port au Prince called Cité Soleil. Driving into St Catherine's Hospital compound is like moving to first class from steerage on a luxury liner. Here you can positively smell foreign aid money. The centre is headed by the Haitian organization, Centres for Development of Health (CDS), under the directorship of Dr Reginald Boulos. In a paper on the centre, Worth Cooley-Prost, a researcher I met in Haiti who was exploring how US foreign aid money was being spent, writes:

Dr Boulos's CDS is by far the most powerful recipient of USAID 'humanitarian' assistance in Haiti. The flagship CDS offices are in Cité Soleil, with other major programmes in Gonaives and Cap Haitien. CDS receives a bewildering tangle of grants, contracts, subcontracts and sub-subcontracts originating with USAID, the NIH, and other US government agencies, amounting to many millions a year. Between those funds, money from the intelligence-linked charity AmeriCares, and some foreign donors, Dr Boulos has controlled a budget larger than the Ministry of Health [Haitian]. USAID has funded medical research in Cité Soleil continuously since 1975.[4]

Cooley-Prost and her colleagues had been making a special investigation into measles vaccine trials in HIV positive babies at this centre. She discovered that over a decade, Haitian infants already enrolled in an ongoing HIV study here, had been given an experimental measles vaccine at 10 to 500 times the usual dose levels. At the time when the original grant proposal for the HIV study at Cité Soleil stated the intention to evaluate measles and another vaccine in HIV positive infants, it was already known that the measles vaccine was associated with lasting immunosuppression.

Some of the babies had been given the vaccine as young as four months, contrary to long-standing WHO recommendations to delay measles vaccination until the age of nine months. Worth Cooley-Prost reported that 'Independent analysis ultimately confirmed that the vaccine caused deaths, particularly in girls, and seemed to cause long-term negative effects on the babies' immune systems. Given these findings the WHO rescinded its recommendation to use the vaccine.'[5] When I visited Cité Soleil I was unaware of the above information. My main intention was to find out if there was or ever had been an AIDS epidemic in Haiti.

At the St Catherine's Hospital we found a quietly spoken woman, Mme Ursule François, the senior nursing officer, whose calm intelligent face told you she had seen most things in life and there were few surprises left. As she chatted, slowly she began to open up. She had seen thousands of cases of TB. She said she saw no difference in the medical picture between patients with TB who were HIV positive and patients with TB who were HIV negative. She thought the whole 'AIDS and Haiti' scene had been exaggerated and believed that hidden agendas were at work.

At the project statistician's office we met Evelyne Leontus. She was concerned about the fear that AIDS plague terror tactics engendered. She said she knew of many people who, when suffering from infections, would not go near a doctor or hospital for fear of being diagnosed HIV positive. She opened her books up for us and we compared figures for HIV testing over a two-year period. We looked at the month of January 1993 and compared it with the month of November 1994. In the first month of 1993, 154 tests were performed and 42 were positive. In November 1994, 250 tests were performed and 78 were positive. 'The more you test, the more you find,' she said.

That seemed to summarize what had happened to AIDS in Haiti: the search for AIDS had indeed uncovered plenty of immuno-deficiency, but no one was willing to consider how the old diseases like TB tend to affect the immune system. So old diseases, now being tested for with new HIV related methods, were acquiring new labels with deadly results. As the saintly Sister Sunupa had said, 'Because we know they will definitely die of AIDS, we have decided we cannot afford to give HIV positive patients medication.'

Chapter 13

Poppers and AIDS: Haemophilia and AIDS

Two Neglected Areas of Research

We once counted over a thousand programmes about AIDS on British and US television; all gave the same old emotive HIV-based story with no scientific analysis. Yet there are two areas of concern that could help us understand what causes the devastating erosion of the immune system we see in AIDS and help us solve the puzzle of AIDS. These have never been brought to the public's attention despite extensive documentation in medical journals. They are:

- the use of poppers or amyl and butyl nitrites as sexual stimulants and their link with Kaposi's sarcoma and other AIDS related conditions; and
- the toxic effect on the immune system of repeated injections of Factor VIII, the coagulant used by haemophiliacs to stop haemorrhaging.

The evidence is there but the will to inquire is blocked by the familiar sense of horror that any challenge to HIV might make young people stop using condoms and might point a finger too directly at the (tiny) proportion of gay men and haemophiliacs who may be at great risk of severe immune suppression.

Poppers: Dangerous Inhalants

The gay scene is very much in denial about what is going on. As a gay man who lives on the scene, I see that the gay scene in London runs on poppers and Ecstasy. The sex scene runs on poppers and the night club scene runs on Ecstasy, coke, speed, acid. So my experience with people with AIDS *is I don't have any clients who do not have what I term a toxic history.*

(Gareth James, homeopath, London)

Their street names are, Rush, Kix, Hardware, Locker Room, Liquid Gold, Rave and many others. They have been widely available in the UK through sex shops, gay bars, pubs, clubs and by mail order. They are emitted through ventilators in discotheques and are used primarily by gay men as a sexual stimulant to dilate the anal orifice. They can enhance and prolong orgasm or produce a 'high' during dancing. They are also mutagenic (that is cause changes in the genetic make-up of a cell structure or can cause the genetic component of cells to change) and they are carcinogenic in animals.[1]

In 1989 poppers became a 'banned hazardous product' in the USA. It is illegal to manufacture, distribute, import or sell any isobutyl nitrite substances or any consumer product 'used for inhaling or otherwise introduced into the body for euphoric or physical effect'. However, the manufacturers of poppers in the USA overcame this hurdle by changing the chemical formula and marketing the resulting products as video head and carburettor cleaners.

Originally, poppers (amyl and butyl nitrites) were used to dilate blood vessels and ease angina pectoris, a heart condition. The name 'poppers' came from the sound of breaking glass when the original small ampoules containing the medicinal liquid were snapped open. But those doses were limited and under medical supervision. Today, you can see young people on the dance floor with an open screw top bottle dangling around their necks as they sniff at will throughout the night.

In the very early days of AIDS, poppers were thought to be an important causal factor. The first 'cluster' of gay men with AIDS in California had all used poppers to assist anal intercourse. Their condition was originally described as GRID – gay related immune deficiency. James

204

Curran and his colleagues at the Centers for Disease Control thought at the time that a 'bad' batch of poppers might be to blame. But as soon as HIV appeared on the scene, the toxic hypothesis was dropped and the virus/AIDS hypothesis was embraced with enthusiasm both by the medical orthodoxy and the gay community. However, John Lauritsen and his colleague Hank Wilson did not let go so easily, 'The evidence against poppers has continued to accumulate,' they wrote.

For several years, major articles in the most prestigious medical journals in the world have discussed the immunosuppressive and other harmful effects of poppers, and their possible role in causing AIDS. The question is no longer whether, but rather how much of a role poppers play in causing AIDS. Are poppers a relatively minor or a very major co-factor? So far as the effect of poppers on health, there is no doubt that they are harmful. For some individuals, even a single episode of snorting poppers can be life-threatening.[2]

Lauritsen and Wilson went on to describe the scientific picture. They pointed to a study comparing two groups of gay men who were HIV antibody positive, one group with symptoms of AIDS and the other not, which demonstrated that usage of nitrite inhalants (poppers) proved to be one of the most important risk factors for developing AIDS, and especially the AIDS defining condition, Kaposi's sarcoma.[3]

Poppers are hazardous to health in many different ways. They damage the immune system, reduce the ability of blood vessels to carry oxygen, cause anaemia and can damage the lungs. They have also been shown to be mutagenic – that is they can cause genes to change, and then the danger is they can develop into a pre-cancerous stage.[4] Organic nitrites, like poppers, are also directly carcinogenic. They can combine with other substances to form deadly cancer-causing compounds known as N-nitroso compounds. In a study by Karl Jorgensen he describes these compounds as having 'the capacity to induce cancer after only one dose'.[5]

Dr Harry Haverkos, working at the US National Institute on Drug Abuse has researched the health hazards of nitrite inhalants over many years. In a 1994 paper for *Environmental Health Perspectives*,[6] he ran through the history of nitrite inhalant abuse.

They began to be bought widely in the United States in the late 1960s by apparently healthy young men. This led the Food and Drug Adminis-tration (FDA) to reinstate a prescription requirement in 1968. As it became more difficult to get hold of poppers for non-medical recreational purposes, they began to be marketed under the guise of 'liquid incense' and 'room odorizers'.

Haverkos focused on two links between poppers and AIDS: the effect of poppers on the immune system and their association with AIDS-related Kaposi's sarcoma:

Nitrite inhalants have been commonly abused substances in the United States. Nitrite inhalants and AIDS was a popular topic in the early 1980s when the cause of AIDS was not known. With the discovery of HIV, concern about nitrite use in the USA waned. However, nitrite inhalant use is asso-ciated with behavioural relapse and HIV transmission among gay men, with decreased lymphocyte counts and natural killer cell activity in a few laboratory studies, and it remains a candidate cofactor in the pathogenesis of AIDS-related Kaposi's sarcoma ... anecdotal reports of increased fre-quency of AIDS-related KS on the chest and face, especially the nose, and in the lungs are consistent with the body areas most heavily exposed to nitrite vapours when inhaled.

Poppers are big business – the biggest money-maker in the gay business world. During the 1970s, gross profits were estimated at $50 million per annum. It is ironic that the world's largest manufacturer of poppers, Great Lakes Products, produced a series of advertisements in 1983, run in gay publications, entitled 'Blueprint for Health'. The advertisements gave advice on how to stay healthy through exercise, nutrition and stress reduction, yet Great Lakes Products was selling a highly toxic substance, which it had to know was used as a recre-ational sex aid by some people in the gay world.

Although poppers were restricted to prescription only more than 20 years' ago in the USA and were subsequently banned altogether, their sale has continued in the UK through sex shops selling them as room odorizers. This led the *News of the World* to campaign against 'the deadly sex drug' and George Galloway to call for a ban on the sale of poppers. Galloway told *Capital Gay* that he was concerned at the prevalence of the use of poppers among gay men, and felt the chemical could have an adverse effect on the immune system of those who are HIV positive. The reply he received in the House of Commons reveals that the Advisory Council had considered a ban on three separate occasions, but maintained that 'although poppers pose a limited health hazard when misused, they are not dependence forming and do not give rise to the sort of social problems which are sufficient to justify their control under the Misuse of Drugs Act.'[7]

The Advisory Council on the Misuse of Drugs must have been badly out of touch because the problem of poppers misuse in adolescents was already worrying many community workers and members of the police. No longer were poppers confined to the gay community, they had become a favourite sniffing drug among school children. By early 1994, the situation had become serious in certain areas. This is how Neil Western of the *Birmingham Post* describes a 13-year-old user, 'It was the excitement John liked – the buzz, the thrill of doing something he was not supposed to. A bit like smoking but more daring. It came in a small brown medicine bottle with a gold wrapper marked, "Not to be taken by children".' 'It was a clear fluid with a pungent smell he was told to sniff and get high on. It worked. He felt good for a few minutes but, then the sickness set in which lasted for hours.'[8]

Pupils as young as 11 were exposed to amyl nitrites in schools, and police in the West Midlands had become worried that poppers were now freely available to schoolchildren but they were powerless to stop the abuse. 'It's no more illegal than eating a chip butty,' said Detective Constable John Crump of the West Midlands Drugs Squad.'[9] North Staffordshire Trading Standards officers also took up the issue as did the MP for Stoke South, George Stevenson, who called for a ban on the sale of poppers in the UK. Others who had been raising the issue for some time in the gay community were Cass Mann from Positively Healthy and his colleague Wayne Moore. They launched a 'Popper Stoppers' campaign to alert and raise awareness of the health risks involved in poppers use, particularly among members of the gay community. Wayne Moore pointed out that attitudes to poppers in the gay community were relaxed and permissive. Poppers were seen to be relatively harmless and their enjoyable effects were considered to out-weigh any health risks. Those who used them in the gay community saw them as just 'a piece of fun' with no long-term consequences.

But it has not all been a one way traffic away from the poppers link to AIDS. The US NIH convened a top level meeting on the subject in May 1994, inviting both Robert Gallo and Peter Duesberg. There was unanimous agreement that poppers were a risk factor in AIDS and even Robert Gallo admitted that there was a high correlation between poppers abuse and Kaposi's sarcoma in gay men and supported the call for further research into the subject.

A major step forward in the UK occurred in 1996 when Sue Sharpe, director of legal services at the Royal Pharmaceutical Society, decided to send representatives to several sex shops in central London secretly to record how the effects of poppers were described by shop assistants. The salesmen in the different sex shops described the effects of pop-pers as producing a 'buzz', a 'rush of blood' and that 'they relax muscles'. These descriptions met with the Medicines Act definition of a medicine, and they were therefore in contravention of the Medicines Act. The Royal Pharmaceutical Society took legal action against one shop, the Zipper Store in London, owned by Millivers (also publishers of the magazine *Gay Times*). Millivers admitted illegally supplying medicines for human consumption and were fined £100.

Since then poppers can only be sold through pharmacies and in January 1997 amyl nitrite was restricted to a prescription only drug. However, sex shops are continuing to sell poppers, asking clients to sign a form confirming that they will be used as room odorizers. Stephen Lutener, head of the inspection and enforcement division at the Royal Pharmaceutical Society told me, 'It's like selling combat knives and saying they are for peeling carrots.'[10]

Haemophilia or Haemophilia/AIDS: Where's the Distinction?

Sue Threakall is one of those capable, tough and reliable Englishwomen who restore one's faith in human nature. She decided to sue Wellcome and her local health authority for causing the death of her husband Bob. It was widely believed that haemophiliacs who tested positive for HIV had been infected by HIV-contaminated Factor VIII, the blood clotting factor they need to inject in order to make their blood coagulate.

Sue's husband Bob, a civil servant, had haemophilia and tested positive for HIV in 1985. However, he had continued to work and, according to Sue, was lively, gregarious and generally well during this period. At this time AZT was prescribed to individuals who were HIV positive and had a low T-cell count but were asymptomatic (had not developed symptoms of AIDS-defining diseases).

In 1989, Bob Threakall was prescribed AZT and from then on things went steadily downhill. There was great enthusiasm among doctors to prescribe AZT to asymptomatic HIV positive people at that time because of the results of the US study purporting to show benefit from the drug in this group of people.[11] The three-year trial, however, had been cut short after only nine months and there was unease among some doctors about the way the trial had been conducted (cf. Dr Michael Lange, Chapter 8). And later on, when the results of the Concorde study emerged showing no benefit in adults taking AZT who had no symptoms of AIDS, Professor Ian Weller (who conducted the Concorde study) openly stated at the Berlin World AIDS Conference that he would not prescribe AZT to such patients.

Sue watched her husband's health swiftly deteriorate once he started taking AZT. It took 18 months for Bob to die. His deterioration was put down to HIV but Sue thought differently. Bob had never been diagnosed as having AIDS-defining symptoms before being put on to AZT. She had seen our film, *AZT: Cause for Concern*, and decided to write to Peter Duesberg. He responded with a batch of papers about AZT's toxicity which he described as 'AIDS by prescription'. This convinced Sue that she must take legal action. Her solicitor, Graham Ross, took up her case and sued Wellcome, the National Institute of Allergy and Infectious Diseases (whose director, Dr Anthony Fauci, headed the AZT trials in asymptomatics), as well as her local health authority (for allowing the drug to be administered). Sue became the first person in history to get legal aid to sue for damages from AZT. Graham Ross decided to home in on her local health authority alone and the case of negligence against it is ongoing. Several other litigants have been added to her case and lawyers in other countries have contacted Ross for assistance on the subject of AZT damage.

Peter Duesberg had been making a careful study of the anomalies involved in the links made between haemophilia and AIDS. He had noted that haemophiliacs with and without HIV were presenting with exactly the same disease patterns. In a paper submitted to the *Lancet* in August 1992, Duesberg outlined his case.[12] (These points were eventually included in Duesberg's larger paper published in *Pharmacology and Therapeutics*.)[13] He pointed out that of the 20,000 haemophiliacs in the USA, about 15,000 (75 per cent) were HIV positive. Of those, only 300 had developed AIDS annually over the previous five years. This amounted to a 2 per cent AIDS risk for American HIV-infected haemophiliacs.

Duesberg's paper published in *Pharmacology and Therapeutics* stated that:

According to the virus-AIDS hypothesis one would have expected that by now (about one 10-year-HIV-latent-period after infection) at least 50 per cent of the 15,000 HIV-positive American haemophiliacs would have developed AIDS or died from AIDS. But the 2 per cent annual AIDS risk indicates that the average HIV-positive haemophiliac would have to wait for 25 years to develop AIDS diseases from HIV, which is the same as their current median age. The median age of American haemophiliacs has increased from 11 years in 1972 to 20 years in 1982 and to over 25 years in 1986, despite the infiltration of HIV in 75 per cent. Thus one could make a logical argument that HIV, instead of decreasing the lifespan of haemophiliacs has in fact increased it.[14]

Duesberg then went on to point out that disease and death in haemophiliacs who are HIV positive is the same as in those who are HIV negative, and that immunodeficiency in haemophiliacs is independent of HIV. Most studies show that lifetime dosage of blood transfusions and Factor VIII lead to the suppression of immunity which in turn leads to diseases categorized within the AIDS definition. Before Factor VIII, most haemophiliacs died as adolescents from internal bleeding.

The introduction of Factor VIII has indeed prolonged their lives, but this long-term transfusion of foreign proteins contained in the donated plasma used for Factor VIII has taken its toll.

Duesberg blamed the long-term transfusion of foreign proteins as the cause of immunodeficiency in haemophiliacs with and without HIV. He also pointed out that if HIV were an infectious, sexually transmitted virus, why did so few wives of haemophiliacs contract AIDS defining diseases? The Centers for Disease Control reported 94 wives of US haemophiliacs with AIDS defining diseases in the seven years between 1985 and 1992.[15] (AIDS defining diseases consist of 29 old diseases like pneumonia, which are only called AIDS if HIV is present.) This simply reflected normal disease and death rates in the general population from those 29 old diseases.[16] Duesberg concluded by saying, 'Since transfusion of foreign proteins appears to cause immunodeficiency in haemophiliacs, the rationale for prescribing the DNA chain terminator AZT as anti-HIV therapy must be reconsidered.'[17]

A study of one cohort of haemophiliacs in Edinburgh, conducted by Dr Christopher Ludlum, has often been held up as an example of why it must be wrong to hold the position that HIV does not cause 'haemophilia/AIDS'.[18] The haemophilia studies in question, when interpreted by Ludlum, purported to show that only HIV positive haemophiliacs in this particular cohort of 32 patients (all of whom had been exposed to the same batch of HIV infected Factor VIII concentrate) progressed to AIDS. None of the HIV negatives progressed to AIDS. When put this way, the evidence is compelling indeed. But the interpretation of these studies needs close examination.

The paper described how, of the 32 patients, 18 'became antibody positive'. The other 14, exposed to the same allegedly HIV contaminated batch of Factor VIII, did not seroconvert. Why these 14 did not become HIV positive is a question the orthodoxy has been unable to answer. The fact remains that they were negative and did not progress to AIDS defining diseases. This study is held up as the great example of why HIV must be the cause of AIDS. Here was proof. None of the HIV negatives progressed to AIDS, only the positives.

So, let us take a closer look at the 18 HIV positive patients. To say that only HIV positives progressed to AIDS is a gross oversimplification of the truth. The fact is that only *some* of the HIV positives progressed to AIDS. In the study, ten of the HIV positives did not progress to AIDS at all. In other words, over half of those infected remained well. Why? Nobody ever talks about them. When you take a closer look at the remaining eight who did progress to AIDS, you see that every single one of those had a particular genetically inherited blood disorder called HLA (human lymphocyte antigen) haplotype A1 B8 DR3. This means that they had an inherited immunological weakness. As the paper itself states, 'The less favourable clinical course is strongly associated with the HLA haplotype A1 B8 DR3,' and continues, 'the general concept that individuals bearing the A1 B8 DR3 haplotype are immunologically hyperactive may have important implications for our understanding of the pathogenesis of AIDS.' An important sentence in the study, which should have been given far greater significance, says, 'We have already noted that the risk of seroconversion after exposure to the contaminated batch of Factor VIII was related to the number of bottles of that batch actually used and to the number of units of Factor VIII used per year.'[19]

The toxic effects of Factor VIII on the immune system and the fact that the AIDS-like diseases occurring in haemophiliacs have been directly linked with the age of the haemophiliac patient and the amount of Factor VIII they had taken, were borne out by the emergence of further studies on the severe immunosuppressive effects of Factor VIII. The original Factor VIII formula consisted of less than 1 per cent of the vital clotting factor. The rest were impurities. The studies now showed a dramatic improvement in the health of haemophiliacs who were given a new purified form of Factor VIII consisting of 99 per cent clotting factor and only 1 per cent impurities.[20]

The new product cost twice as much as the old one, raising the average cost of treatment to between £12,000 and £14,000 a year and up to £50,000 for heavy users, so it was only made available to haemophiliacs who had been diagnosed HIV positive (thereby establishing a two-tier system favouring HIV positive haemophiliacs). When asked for his opinion of these findings, Professor Gordon Stewart said they were immensely important:

If this work is confirmed it means that patients may not get AIDS at all. It also gives us an immense clue to the mechanism of AIDS. We now know that if the haemophiliacs are infused with the impure concentrates, they get changes that resemble AIDS; and if they get the high purity product, they don't get those changes. So the probability is that haemophiliacs' response is to the foreign protein in their treatment, and not to HIV. The allegation that haemophiliac patients get AIDS because of being infected by HIV has to be questioned.[21]

Someone else who had come to question the links between HIV and haemophilia was Russell Schoch, editor of *California Monthly*, the alumni magazine at the University of California, Berkeley. He had been following the arguments closely and had published two expositions of the anti-HIV arguments with great clarity.[22] Schoch's son had haemophilia. In a moving piece taking up a whole page of *Newsweek* called 'Dad, I'm HIV positive', Schoch writes, 'Both my son and I strongly support the effort to re-examine the hypothesis that HIV causes AIDS, a hypothesis that has yet to save a single human life.'[23]

By now the conviction that haemophiliacs who were HIV positive had been contaminated by HIV infected blood in their Factor VIII clotting agents had led to a mass of litigation. By the end of 1990, in the UK over 1000 adults and 175 children were claiming compensation for having allegedly been infected by contaminated Factor VIII. The British government decided to add an extra £42 million to the initial total of £34 million made as an *ex-gratia* payment earlier in the year. In Europe and America new claims for compensation were flooding in every day.

At the Royal Hospital in Perth, Western Australia, biophysicist Eleni Eleopulos was thinking differently. She had been working steadily with her hospital colleague, Valendar Turner and also with her long-term colleagues David Causer, and Professor John Papadimitriou, head of the department of pathology, University of Western Australia. Together, they had become convinced that HIV could not possibly be in Factor VIII, let alone actually reproduce itself and go on to infect other cells. They prepared an article for a special edition of the journal *Genetica* with the following bold and unambiguous abstract:

In this review, the association between the Acquired Immune Deficiency Syndrome (AIDS) and haemophilia has been carefully examined, especially the data that have been interpreted as indicating transmission of the human immunodeficiency virus (HIV) to the recipients of purportedly contaminated Factor VIII preparations. In our view, the published data do not prove the hypothesis that such transmission occurs, and therefore HIV cannot account for AIDS in haemophiliacs.[24]

This special edition of *Genetica* had been handed over to Peter Duesberg to edit by its editor-in-chief, John McDonald, Professor of Genetics at Athens University, Georgia. In his foreword McDonald mentions that a claimed:

de facto *conspiracy exists within the scientific community to prevent dissenting views and alternative AIDS hypotheses from being presented to the scientific and general public. . . . Ignoring charges of scientific censorship can only work to undermine the public's confidence not only in the prevailing scientific view but also in the entire scientific establishment. In providing this forum for alternative AIDS hypotheses,* Genetica *hopes to dispel the notion that a 'conspiracy of silence' exists within the scientific community.*[25]

Is There Any HIV in Factor VIII?

This important journal allowed Eleopulos and her colleagues to address some of the fundamental issues surrounding haemophilia and AIDS, and to raise questions that had never been allowed into print before. Questions like: Why is it that HIV has never actually been isolated from Factor VIII? How could HIV survive the freezing, thawing and sterilization by filtration process involved in the manufacture of Factor VIII? Why is it that there are no cases of AIDS/haemophilia involving KS (Kaposi's sarcoma) when this was regarded as one of the key AIDS defining diseases? Why do the CDCs have documented cases of haemophilia/AIDS that are HIV negative, with no indicator diseases? How can it be that 'HIV' is claimed to have been 'isolated' from children with haemophilia who had no other risk factors and where their Factor VIII had been checked and rechecked and found negative for

HIV antibodies? 'This is as close a proof as one can get,' writes Eleopoulos, 'that what has been called HIV infection in haemophiliacs is not caused by an exogenous retrovirus to which haemophiliacs have been exposed but by the administration of Factor VIII preparations.'[26]

For cell-free HIV viral particles (particles that have not integrated themselves into another cell's DNA) to be able to go on and infect other cells they have to have an envelope protein called gp120 on their outer shell. These proteins form the projecting knobs on the viral particles that are said to be crucial for HIV to be able to latch on to and infect another cell. Eleopulos focuses, in her article, on the fact that HIV simply could not survive the process of manufacture of Factor VIII and that even if cell-free viral particles did get through, they could not constitute a meaningful source of HIV transmission. In other words, they would not be capable of going on to infect new cells because they were no more than incomplete pieces of viral debris without the necessary gp120 knobs on their protein coats.

Eleopulos points out that in 1983 Gallo himself said, 'The viral envelope which is required for infectivity is very fragile. It tends to come off when the virus buds from infected cells, thus rendering the particles incapable of infecting new cells.' Having admitted this, how could Gallo explain a way in which HIV could infect new cells? As always, he had an answer at the ready. He said that without the viral envelope, infection *may* require 'cell to cell contact'.[27] This cell to cell contact would do away with the need for a protein coat. However, Eleopulos concludes that since gp120, said to be crucial to HIV's ability to infect new cells, is not found in cell free particles, then even if HIV particles are present in plasma or Factor VIII preparations, they will not be infectious. Recent research confirms that over 99 per cent of HIV viral particles extruded by cells are defective and described by the orthodoxy itself as non infectious particles.[28]

Factor VIII and False Positive HIV Test Results

Eleopulos then goes on to tackle the issue of false positive HIV antibody tests in people with haemophilia. She points out that the presence of antibodies to HIV in people with haemophilia may not mean that they are true positives. She quotes Dr Philip Mortimer, director of the Virus Reference Laboratory of the Public Health Laboratory Service (PHLS) in London:

Diagnosis of HIV infection is based almost entirely on detection of antibodies to HIV, but there can be misleading cross-reactions between HIV-1 antigens [the proteins said to provoke an HIV antibody response] and antibodies formed against other antigens, and these may lead to false-positive reactions. Thus, it may be impossible to relate an antibody specifically to HIV-1 infection [emphasis in original].[29]

In other words, antibodies made after an influenza vaccination could react in an HIV test and make it appear that HIV, instead of the influenza antigen, is present.

Then came the real bombshell. Eleopulos says that a significant number of AIDS patients will have a false positive HIV antibody test because haemophiliacs, gay men and intravenous drug users are all subjected to a wide variety of foreign antigens and infectious agents that are not specific to HIV. She goes on to describe how most haemophiliacs were tested for HIV before 1988 with the ELISA test. (Only very few were confirmed with a Western blot test in those days.) She says there is a distinct possibility that if haemophiliacs tested only with ELISA or even with ELISA and Western blot before 1988 were reappraised, a significant number would no longer be classified as HIV positive. Think of the implications! All HIV positive haemophiliacs, in fact all HIV positives period, tested before 1988 should be recalled for retesting, and all the litigation surrounding contaminated Factor VIII would have to be reassessed.

Antibodies 'Identifying' HIV are not Specific to HIV

The paper then attacks the very basis of the identification of HIV. Protein 24 (p24) is one of the key proteins said to be specific to HIV. Eleopulos demonstrates, by a search through the literature, that p24 is not proved to be specific to retroviruses and cannot be specific to HIV because the p24 of other retroviruses elicits the same antibodies.

It is interesting to note here that although Gallo and Montagnier, in a joint publication, claimed that p24 is unique to HIV, Gallo has repeatedly stated that the p24 of HIV, and of two other human retroviruses, which he claims to have isolated from humans, can immunologically cross-react. In other words, p24 cannot be specific to HIV.[30] Eleopoulos quotes several examples to back this up. The allegedly all-important p24 has been found in a high proportion of 'indeterminate' or HIV negative blood donors[31] and it appears in the blood of previously HIV negative patients, after receiving transfusions of blood that had been tested and found to be HIV negative.[32] It has also been detected in up to 36 per cent of patients with SLE (systemic lupus erythematosus)[33] and in patients who have received organ transplants. In most cases the p24 disappeared a few months after the transplant.

Eleopulos then makes her first hint at the fact that HIV, or the proteins that are claimed to identify HIV, may not be specific to HIV at all, and simply proteins that are in all of us (endogenous) and only flare up when the body is under severe immunological stress – that HIV may have been wrongly identified, that in fact HIV may not exist at all. She proposes that there are many reasons why the p24 (said to identify HIV) detected in the blood of haemophiliacs and organ recipients, after being cultured in the laboratory, may not be HIV at all. They may instead be either non-viral protein or the protein of an endogenous retrovirus. She concludes this section of her paper by flatly stating that what has been called HIV infection in haemophiliacs '*is not caused by an exogenous retrovirus to which haemophiliacs have been exposed through Factor VIII*' (emphasis added).[34]

So what is making haemophiliacs ill? Eleopulos quotes many reports that describe how the impure Factor VIII product itself is considered to cause immune abnormalities like a low T4 cell count and general immune suppression, even when produced from a population of blood donors not at risk for AIDS. She also points out that AIDS-like diseases (atypical pneumonias, including pneumocystis carinii pneumonia – PCP) in an appreciable number of haemophiliacs were reported before the AIDS era. The paper concludes by reminding us of the impurities in Factor VIII and how haemophilia AIDS cases are directly related to the quantity of Factor VIII product haemophiliacs have taken (dose-related) and the length of time they have taken it for (age related).

The final footnote to her paper is of crucial importance, and features as a 'note added in proof'. Since the Perth group completed its paper for *Genetica,* the Centers for Disease Control forwarded a copy of its fact sheet (CDC 1994) on HIV transmission. In this they state quite openly: 'CDC studies have shown that drying of even these high concentrations of HIV reduces the number of infectious viruses [in the Factor VIII] by 90 to 99 per cent within several hours ... drying of HIV infected human blood or other body fluids reduces the theoretical risk of environmental transmission to that which has been observed – essentially zero." Commenting on the fact sheet, Eleopulos et al. state: 'It is thus inexplicable, given their own data, that the CDC continues to regard patients with haemophilia at risk of HIV infection via contaminated Factor VIII concentrates and enigmatic that another explanation for 'HIV' and AIDS in haemophiliacs has not been sought.'[35]

The Obstinate Community of the Unconvinced

Duesberg and Eleopulos's challenge to the virus/AIDS hypothesis through their critical analysis of the anomalies in haemophilia/AIDS, had not escaped the AIDS orthodoxy. Sooner or later they would have to respond. And respond they did, in September 1995, with the publication in *Nature* of a letter from Sarah Darby et al. analysing death rates in haemophiliacs before and after HIV 'infection'.[36] The letter was accompanied by a ringing editorial from John Maddox and a decidedly pointed press release from the MRC. The article claimed that the death rate in haemophiliacs in the seven years between 1985 and 1992 was ten times greater in those haemophiliacs infected with HIV. (It should be remembered that AZT therapy for HIV-positive haemophiliacs was introduced after 1987.)

Maddox began his editorial by saying that the letter was a further reason for discretion on the part of those who hold that HIV has nothing or little to do with the cause of AIDS. Then he went even further, 'Those who have made the running in the long controversy over HIV in AIDS, Dr Peter Duesberg of Berkeley, California, in particular, have a heavy responsibility that can only be discharged by a public acknowledgement of error, honest or otherwise. And the sooner the better.' However, Maddox did acknowledge the following flaws in Darby's work, 'Yet it is safe to predict that there will be complaints from the obstinate community of the unconvinced that Darby et al. have failed to provide full details of the drug regimen followed by the 6000 people on the register, and that until they do, their conclusion has no force.'[37]

The MRC press release had no reservations. It crowed, 'Details of a 15-year study of Britain's haemophiliacs released today show that the big rise in deaths over the last ten years is caused by HIV infection. Researchers believe their results should silence critics who argue that HIV is not the cause of AIDS.'[38]

The Darby haemophilia study also gave Steve Connor another opportunity to twist his dagger into the AIDS dissidents. 'The world's largest study of haemophiliacs has proven categorically that HIV causes AIDS, a link disputed by a small number of maverick scientists who enjoyed extensive publicity in Britain ... the new research is seen as the final refutation of the views of Peter Duesberg.'[39] Duesberg swiftly penned his response. He composed a 1500-word article with 19 references for the *Lancet*. In it he rejected Darby's findings and concentrated on his view that the immunosuppressive effects of foreign proteins contaminating Factor VIII and the toxic effects of AZT, given to HIV positive haemophiliacs, accounted for the AIDS/haemophilia deaths.

Richard Horton, the recently appointed editor of the *Lancet*, who had previously lent a very sympathetic ear to the dissident debate, turned Duesberg's article down but asked for a 500-word letter with no more than five references, which he duly published in November 1995.[40] In customary adversarial style, Duesberg issued a challenge to Horton in his letter. He said he was willing to concede if Horton could prove him wrong in two predictions. This first prediction was that if two groups of haemophiliacs were to be studied who were matched for their lifetime consumption of Factor VIII and all medications, but one group was HIV positive and one negative, they would prove to have identical AIDS risks.

The second prediction was that if two groups of HIV positive haemophiliacs were to be studied, matched for lifetime dosage of Factor VIII, but one group was treated with AZT and other anti-AIDS drugs and the other not, then the drug treated group would prove to have a ten times higher mortality rate than the untreated group.[41] To this day, this research has never been undertaken. Now it was Eleni Eleopuos's turn to respond to the Darby study. She sent a powerful rebuttal to *Nature* which was rejected. Then Huw Christie and his co-editor Molly Ratcliffe took up the issue in their magazine *Continuum* and published a press release saying:

Far from apologizing as called for in an editorial in Nature *accompanying the present study, we 'the obstinate community of the unconvinced' have every reason to remain so, and consider that the study simply supports the views held by Professor Duesberg (Berkeley), Eleni Papadopulos Eleopulos (Perth), Dr Harvey Bialy (New York) and others that HIV is not the cause of AIDS. ... On the contrary, we hereby request and require that the scientists involved readopt proper scientific principles in this very important field of public health.*[42]

The following issue of *Continuum* then published Eleopulos's rejected paper in full. In it, she and her colleagues pointed out that the claim by Darby et al. that the 85 per cent increase in death rate among HIV positive haemophiliacs was due to HIV could only be sustained if the study had evidence to show that the cause of the extra deaths in HIV positive group was AIDS. In fact, 168 (over half) of the 403 HIV positive deaths were from causes other than AIDS, and the ones claimed to have died from AIDS and HIV were misleading because AIDS is constituted from more than 25 different diseases and because no single infectious agent has ever been found to cause so many distinct and unrelated diseases.[43]

The obstinate community of the unconvinced was growing apace in London. Now it was girding itself for the next phase and *Continuum* proved an important forum at this moment in the story of AIDS dissent for the arguments from a young virologist in Germany, Dr Stefan Lanka, from a group of retired scientists in Switzerland headed by Professor Alfred Hässig, and from the team in Perth that had inspired them – arguments to show that HIV itself does not exist.

Chapter 14

Does HIV Exist?

Buenos Aires AIDS Conference: The Growing Doubts

I sat back in the comfortable first-class seat of the Boeing 747 and peered down at the vast expanse of Atlantic Ocean, *en route* to Buenos Aires courtesy of the Argentine Ministry of Health. How had I got here?

It was all thanks to the herculean efforts of Dr Ricardo Leschot, an Argentine doctor working in the field of AIDS, who had been making big waves in Argentina. On many radio and television interviews he had announced his heresy – that HIV did not cause AIDS. Dr Leschot had noticed that many of his AIDS patients had fallen apart before his very eyes under the devastating strain of living with the HIV death sentence, and under the toxic effects of AZT. Leschot had worked with several of them, managed to talk them through their crisis and persuaded them to come off AZT. He had seen some of them begin to thrive again. At the very least there was a need to challenge established assumptions. This inspired him to organize an international conference on AIDS in April 1995 to which he had invited as many AIDS dissidents as he could. The conference was to generate a few sparks, for many of the delegates had arrived from provincial towns in Argentina, full of 'HIV awareness' zeal. They were amazed to hear so many speakers challenge the virus/AIDS hypothesis.

Has HIV Ever Been Isolated?

The most dramatic contribution to the conference was provided by German virologist Stefan Lanka. When, a few months earlier, Stefan Lanka had walked into our offices in London brandishing a manuscript in German claiming that HIV did not exist, Hector Gildemeister took a deep breath and thought 'not more of the same only now in German'. Then, when he began to read Lanka's story, he decided this was far from more of the same. It explained many of the question marks to do with HIV. Gildemeister began translating and reshaping the paper for the lay reader. The article took many weeks of toing and froing between himself and Lanka before it was ready and when 'HIV: reality or artefact?' emerged, our world was once again turned upside down.[1]

Stefan Lanka had studied virology at the University of Konstanz in Germany where he had written a doctorate on a marine virus study. He knew a thing or two about virus isolation, for his work had led him to analyse some marine viruses that had never been identified before. He became the first person to isolate two new marine viruses and had a brilliant career ahead of him in the world of orthodox virology – that is until he came across AIDS and the questions that challenged the virus/AIDS hypothesis.

In their paper, 'Is a positive Western blot proof of HIV infection?', Eleni Eleopulos and her team had already pointed out that the proteins said to be specific to HIV could be found in all of us and that the HIV test and related science had to be reappraised.[2] Eleopulos questioned the isolation of HIV and quoted the US Centers for Disease Control saying as far back as 1988 that there was no correlation between the presence of HIV in laboratory cultures and in humans. Influenced by Eleopulos's work, Lanka began to wonder not only whether HIV caused AIDS, but whether HIV even existed at all. After all, he reasoned, it had never been isolated nor reliably photographed; only the proteins said to be specific to HIV were used to report its existence and there had never been a reliable HIV test. The scientific validity of these tests had not been established and the magnitude of inter-laboratory variations between them had not been measured. Test results required interpretation, and the criteria for their interpretation varied not only from laboratory to laboratory but also from month to month.[3]

Here, in Buenos Aires, Lanka went on stage with his own set of props as a mock demonstration kit and, in accomplished style, explained how a retrovirus like HIV could be said to exist through culturing in laboratory dishes and through the test procedures. The identification of HIV, he told his audience, relied on a totally artificial situation, which depended on keeping permanent cell lines going in which HIV was incubated, and using manipulation techniques that turned the cells into no more than a laboratory artefact. These methods were self-perpetuating and wrong. HIV, he announced, has never been isolated and does not even exist. This was bold stuff. It certainly did not sit easily with those HIV sceptics who discounted the HIV/AIDS hypothesis but accepted the existence of the retrovirus as a benign passenger. But Lanka pressed on.

What the prevailing orthodoxy described as the retrovirus HIV had to be incubated in permanent cell lines. These are sometimes called immortalized cell lines and are usually cancer cell lines that continue to replicate unceasingly and allow the HIV cultures to grow in them. So, to 'find' HIV, Gallo and Montagnier had to culture HIV from a patient's blood in the laboratory. Their pronouncements that they could see HIV killing other cells was therefore made from their observation of these cultures, in an environment removed from the body's own immune responses.

Furthermore, Lanka pointed out that to achieve 'HIV activity' these cell lines had to be treated with chemical agents to activate the cells and cause them to divide. The agents would never be encountered in the human body; thus, this was an artificial way of stimulating a response. Using his stage props, Lanka showed how this artificial procedure is referred to as stressing a cell, causing small pieces (never the whole) of RNA to convert into corresponding DNA through the chemical activity of the enzyme reverse transcriptase. This, he said with a flourish, is how retroviruses are said to exist, and how HIV was born.

But, Lanka continued, these are not retroviruses, they are no more than unrelated pieces of RNA that have been transcribed into DNA with the help of the enzyme reverse transcriptase. This chemical activity could sometimes result in the linking together of random pieces of DNA (template switching). In other words, having transcribed one sequence, the reverse transcriptase could transcribe another random piece of RNA and tack it on. 'It's like selecting random words out of a book,' says Lanka, 'constructing a new sentence from them, and then claiming the sentence came from the book.' Lanka's position was that the reverse transcriptase activity and the resulting pieces of DNA said to identify HIV were not specific to HIV. They were a feature of every form of life and were used to repair chromosomal damage. He maintained that the procedures used to 'find' retroviral activity were a construct. They were a device whereby a retroviral activity was identified 'by proxy', and that retroviruses had never been proved actually to exist.

The existence of retroviruses, said Lanka, was perpetuated by a group of scientists who 25 years ago misinterpreted the significance of the role of reverse transcriptase. The permanent cell lines these scientists had to manipulate to produce what they called HIV originated from a single laboratory source, were frozen and sent to colleagues around the world who unsurprisingly obtained similar results. These were then held up to be proof of the validity of the existence of retroviruses and the science of retrovirology as a whole. The results, he said, were reproduced over and over again, using the same manipulated cell lines with everyone working from the same originally constructed laboratory phenomenon.[4]

It is crucial to Lanka's case that no photographs of HIV exist, although many a 'photograph' has been published bearing that caption. The truth is that what we are being presented with are not photographs of one virus but of a series of black and white electronmicrographs of separate virus-like particles present in cell cultures (where several types of particles are present) and some are arbitrarily said to be HIV. By juxtaposing these still photographs they can then be made to appear in sequence to represent a real-time event – penetrating a cell, budding out and so forth. This is no more than an animation technique worthy of Walt Disney.

Harvey Bialy, himself a leading AIDS dissident, was not convinced by Lanka. He held firmly to his position that HIV was not the cause of AIDS, but that HIV *had* been isolated. He said Lanka's arguments were esoteric, that they would undermine efforts to show how AIDS science had been wrong about HIV and that they should not be shared with journalists present at the conference. The fact is that even the dissident position on AIDS moves on and the scientific arguments need continual reappraisal proving how fertile was the ground for curiosity and inquiry at the cutting edge of the AIDS debate. The build-up to Lanka's speech in Buenos Aires had been underway for many months. The lines of communication between Lanka, the Eleopulos group in Perth, the Hässig group in Berne and the London dissidents had been busy indeed.

To set Lanka's Buenos Aires speech in its proper context and to understand from where the proteins that are identified as HIV are coming, we need to take a careful look at the work of Eleopulos and Hässig.

The Mechanism of AIDS: Acquired Immune Overload

Every morning Alfred Hässig meets up with his colleagues, a group of retirees in their seventies, in an office in central Berne. They have formed the Study Group on Nutrition and Immunity and, feeling they have all the time in the world now that they are no longer in the professional rat race, meticulously pick apart many of the assumptions in newly emergent fields of science. AIDS has come under their critical eye and, together with Drs Liang Wen-Xi and K. Stampfli (and more recently Dr Heinrich Kremer), they have produced more than 15 papers, some of them published in international journals, challenging the infectious virus/AIDS hypothesis.

Hässig is an experienced immunologist who, for 37 years, was head of the Swiss Red Cross Blood Transfusion Service. Through the series of papers prepared with his colleagues, Hässig has conducted a detailed analysis of the mechanism that causes the immune system breakdown, described as AIDS.[5] In his and his group's opinion, AIDS is the result of a persistent stress response, shifting the metabolism of the body into a state of assault on the immune system which the body cannot sustain (called catabolism). This metabolic situation corresponds with a chronic whole body inflammation, including an accumulation of inflammatory cells, causing antibodies to be formed against proteins from the body's own cells. These are the antibodies that have become confused with anti-HIV antibodies.

The orthodoxy's central argument is that HIV kills the immune system's T-cells (also described as CD4 cells). Says Hässig, 'To state that HIV kills CD4 cells is the biggest mistake in the HIV/AIDS hypothesis.

The AIDS syndrome is caused by a stress response. This is clearly seen in all AIDS patients.' Hässig believes that persistent stress is characterized by an inflammatory response involving the neuroendocrine system. This is described as a hypercortisol state, when the body is forced into producing abnormal amounts of cortisol. 'It is a neuroendocrine condition not a viral one and rightly the concern of immunologists not virologists.'

Hässig points out that Anthony Fauci, the doyen of AIDS research, linked the stress response to AIDS in 1974, ten years before HIV was announced to be the cause of AIDS. His paper showed that cortisol injected into healthy human individuals in order to induce a stress response produced the same depletion of the CD4 group of T-cells (immune system cells) as observed in people with AIDS.[6] 'Isn't it odd', says Hässig, 'that Fauci should have conveniently forgotten his own papers, when HIV reached centre stage?'

Aware that when the body is stressed it produces high levels of antibodies (which are proteins), Hässig began to inquire into the nature of antibodies said to be specific to HIV.[7] He highlighted the fact that patients with the inflammatory autoimmune condition known as SLE (systemic lupus erythematosus) often test positive for HIV antibodies. In a study conducted in 1994, 43 per cent of lupus patients had tested HIV antibody positive.[8] Hässig concluded that the proteins the body was making in these conditions were autoantibodies, which had nothing to do with HIV, but nonetheless tested positive on the HIV test. In other words, what was being found was a raised antibody profile, but these antibodies were not specific to HIV.

But why does the body react against itself and produce these autoantibodies? Hässig explains that every day, apart from making new cells, the body has to remove 1000 million cell particles it no longer needs. These particles may produce RNA and DNA. When the body is under stress it produces even more of these particles. The body's immune defences cannot always recognize all of this material as its own. It loses its ability to differentiate 'self' from 'non-self' (proteins entering the body) and 'altered self' (abnormal proteins made in the body). This is a classic autoimmune response. Lupus (SLE) is not the only condition that can trigger this response. Other autoimmune conditions like arthritis, and diseases like TB, parasites, leprosy, malaria and multiple sclerosis can all produce the same effect. 'We are really at the point', says Hässig, 'where we can recognize the HIV hypothesis for the failure that it is.'

Given the above, Hässig is entirely opposed to the use of AZT. His group has denounced its use and drawn attention to the damage it can cause to the intestines as well as to bone marrow, not to mention to the mitochondria, the vestigial bacteria that have evolved with us to become the vital 'power packs' of human cells. These form the principal energy source of all cells in our body except cancerous cells.[9]

So what can be done to bring an overstressed body back into balance? The Berne group's work on nutrition says that, first, the source of psychological stress and harmful drug therapy must be eliminated, and then action must be taken to control the inflammatory response in the body – this hyperactivation of the immune system producing the proliferation of autoantibodies. This can be helped by reducing the raised oxygen free radicals in the blood. These are incomplete atoms that range around the body causing inflammation and damage.[10] They can be reduced through the intake of vegetable-based antioxidants in plant preparations,[11] and foods like green tea, fresh fruit and tofu, all of which contain antioxidant agents like polyphenols flavonoids and tannins.[12]

One of the main accepted ill-effects of AZT is its damage to the lining of the stomach – causing severe diarrhoea and vomiting. This in turn affects the way the body absorbs nutrients, but the virus/AIDS hypothesis and its attendant drug therapies have left little room for exploring alternative ways of regenerating the immune system and reconstituting the gut.[13] The work of the Berne group is of importance because it is studying practical ways of treating people with immunodeficiency through changes in lifestyle and diet rather than through a cocktail of antiviral drugs.

Meanwhile, as far away as Western Australia, the small group of scientists led by biophysicist Eleni Eleopulos at the Royal Hospital in Perth had continued with its rigorous analysis of the current AIDS orthodoxy – the analysis which had led to the Lanka speech on that Buenos Aires stage. Not only had they produced the important work on haemophilia described in the previous chapter, they had now completed a startling paper challenging the whole basis of the Western blot HIV test.[14] The HIV antibody test does not detect a virus. It tests for antibodies that react with an assortment of proteins, which we are told are unique to HIV. The routine procedure worldwide (except for England since 1992) for testing for HIV has been to perform a double ELISA (enzyme-linked immunosorbent assay) test to check the level of allegedly HIV specific antibodies, and further confirm with a Western blot test.

The ELISA test involves incubating a sample of blood serum with a mixture of the 'HIV specific' proteins. The ELISA is positive if the solution changes colour to a certain density, thereby indicating a reaction between the proteins in the test kit and the patient's antibodies. Because the ELISA is not specific, and can react to non HIV-generated antibodies, most testing authorities strive to eliminate 'false positives' by repeating the ELISA test and carrying out a different further test called the Western blot.[15] The Western blot test is supposed to be able to find which of the HIV proteins are present by identifying antibodies to them. This shows up in a series of bands identifying the presence of a specific set of antibody/protein reactions. The Western blot test has turned out to be so unreliable for HIV diagnosis that the PHLS Virus Reference Laboratory in Britain no longer use it and rely only on the ELISA test. Test results are reached, ideally, through a process of multiple sampling which involves running several ELISA tests on one sample and then sending it for confirmation to another laboratory using a different test kit. However, Western blot is still used as a confirmatory test in most countries around the world. Different countries have different criteria for the number of bands on the Western blot test that are required in order to declare a test HIV positive.

Eleopulos's paper was the scientific confirmation for that groundbreaking speech of Stefan Lanka's in Buenos Aires. Not only did she describe why the proteins said to be specific to HIV were not unique to HIV, but also that even if antibodies to these proteins did show up, they could not be assumed to be a sign of HIV infection. Eleopulos criticized both the ELISA and the Western blot tests. The ELISA antibody test, she said, could only be meaningful when it was standardized, that is when a given test result had the same meaning in all patients, in all laboratories and in all countries. But this was not the case and results remained variable because there was no absolute standard.

To illustrate how the Western blot test was not reproducible she described the Transfusion Safety Study conducted in the USA.[16] Here four samples of blood were put through a quality control procedure and tested with both ELISA and Western blot. Two were declared HIV positive and two negative. These were then submitted for Western blot testing over and over again, sometimes up to 70 times to three different reference laboratories. The results showed some remarkable variations, with the same HIV positive sample coming up positive in one laboratory on three protein bands seven times, and at the same laboratory, on only one band five times. At another laboratory, the same sample produced no bands at all. By the same token, the HIV negative samples produced positive results several times over. Because the decision as to whether or not an individual is HIV positive depends on whether a certain number of required bands are present, this lack of correlation between one laboratory and another is, to say the least, disturbing.

The results of these repeated assays are too detailed to go into in depth, but not only did they vary dramatically within one laboratory and from one laboratory to another, but also the criteria for declaring them positive or negative would have varied from one country to another. Dr Val Turner in Perth made a study of the different criteria.[17] In Australia, for example, at least four protein bands are required, in Canada and much of the USA three or more and across Africa two will do. So all an African has to do is be retested in Australia where he or she might be found negative.

In other words, individuals can be HIV positive or negative depending on which laboratory or test kit or in which country they were tested. Small wonder that Dr Philip Mortimer, head of the PHLS Virus Reference Laboratory in London, has abandoned the use of Western blot testing in the UK. In a quality assessment exercise he found that, 'participating laboratories had developed 11 different sets of criteria to read Western blots. Confusion of this sort must lead to errors,' he wrote.[18]

Eleopulos explained another example of the disturbing anomalies surrounding Western blot in a letter to the *Lancet*. She reminds us of the four women in Sydney who were found to be HIV positive after *in vitro* fertilization with HIV positive semen. This was used by the orthodoxy as one of the clearest demonstrations that AIDS could be spread heterosexually by semen. (None of the women's breast-fed babies became positive.) These four women's diagnoses were based on Western blot tests conducted in 1985 when only one or two bands were required to test positive. Under present criteria, for a positive Western blot in Australia none of the four women or even the donor would be considered HIV positive. 'Neither would any be positive under the criteria set by the FDA and the American Red Cross. In fact, two of the women would not be positive by any criteria anywhere in the world.'[19]

Turner illustrates the flaws in testing by quoting a study of 1.2 million applicants for US military service.[20] Their first ELISA HIV test produced 12,000 positives but only 2000 of these were ultimately shown to be Western blot positive and thus, according to the authors, HIV infected. Writes Turner, 'This left 10,000 positive ELISAs which must have reacted for reasons other than "HIV antibodies", a fitting testimonial to the problem caused by cross-reacting antibodies. ... What this means is that you are not necessarily infected with what your antibodies appear to tell you.' Turner sums up by saying, 'It is proper for a disinterested scientist to allow for the possibility that there are no real HIV antibodies whatsoever, that they are all pretenders.'[21] And finally, when 2210 individuals with syphilis were tested in the USA, 24 per cent tested false positive on ELISA. Of the ten samples that tested repeatedly positive on ELISA, nine were negative on Western blot and, according to the researchers, there was therefore only one 'true positive'.[22]

Eleopulos and her team in Perth have produced a substantial body of work, yet the virological establishment has chosen to ignore her paper on Western blot and its sequel questioning the isolation of HIV.[23] I have heard it said that no matter how right you are, until over 50 per cent of the scientific establishment says you are right, you will be ignored. In the past, however, it was easier to air your view and have your challenging hypothesis put to the test. The nightmare of modern science is that big money, advertising revenues in science journals, drug and test kit patents mean that a challenge to the prevailing orthodoxy is in danger of never being heard – and that heretical point of view may be the right one.

At the conference in Buenos Aires, Lanka told his audience that it was the work of Eleopulos that had led him to go a step further and investigate the use of another way of 'finding HIV' called polymerase chain reaction (PCR). The discovery of this technique by Kary Mullis earned him the Nobel prize for chemistry. He found a way of amplifying DNA so that one could, so to speak, 'find a needle in a haystack'. Where the target DNA is scarcely detectable, the amount may be amplified, thus doubling and redoubling it until a sufficient measurable quantity is available. This technique has been used by AIDS researchers to 'find' HIV and provide proof of massive viral load in AIDS patients. But some critics maintain that what is being found are small fragments of defective viral particles or endogenous particles that do not have sufficient genetic information to reproduce themselves, let alone go on to infect other cells (see Chapter 13).

In Buenos Aires, Lanka went further by saying that these were not even viral particles but stretches of DNA that could be manipulated to give an HIV positive result. Illustrating his point through a series of slides, he described how by shifting only slightly the start point of the primers used for PCR testing, even an HIV negative blood sample can be made to show a positive result. He said he could make even the Archbishop of Canterbury test positive by PCR. This was because, as Eleopulos had pointed out, the genetic identification of the proteins said to be specific to HIV are in all of us and can be tweaked into existence through laboratory manipulation.

So what does this all mean? It means that we must radically alter our thinking about the identification of HIV itself. This position Duesberg finds unacceptable. He believes that the identification of HIV, based on the process of molecular cloning – through which it is claimed that exactly the same HIV structures have been identified independently in different laboratories – is definitive proof that HIV exists and that retroviruses as a whole exist.[24] This is not so, protests Lanka, because the definition of the proteins specific to HIV has never been examined. It was simply announced by Gallo and then confirmed by several of

his colleagues, who unquestioningly accepted Gallo's formula for identifying this new and allegedly catastrophic retrovirus.

Having come so far, we now had a rumbling volcano in the midst of
the once close-knit AIDS dissident community. Duesberg's final words
on this were, 'It seems tragic that over 99 per cent of AIDS researchers
study a virus that does not cause AIDS and that the few who don't are
now engaged in a debate over the existence of a virus that does not
cause AIDS.'[25]

Positively False: HIV Wrongly Identified

It was time to investigate more closely the implications of what was
being said. We decided to home in on the issue of HIV testing. Could
this be a way of providing positive proof of the existence or not of HIV?
The false positive results and the inconsistencies between one test kit
and another and between different laboratories were already providing
strong indications that something was seriously wrong. There are
18,000 people who have been declared HIV positive in the UK. Given
the changes in criteria for diagnosing a positive result, and the accepted
cross-reactions that could cause a 'false positive' result, could it be that
many of these have been wrongly diagnosed?

We were not the only ones to be worrying. Dr Philip Mortimer, at
the PHLS Virus Reference Laboratory in London, said to one of our
researchers in April 1996 that the issues of standards for HIV testing
was 'one of considerable arguments that are not entirely reconcilable.
... We are all very concerned about how specific the tests have been
over ten years now, and this is a cause of great anxiety to us.'
Mortimer was particularly worried about the fact that although he had
laid down guidelines for testing, and was trying to establish a single
agreed policy, 'independent scientists don't want to follow our
reference laboratory guidelines.'[26]

There are many published articles in the medical literature docu-
menting cross-reactions with the HIV test and false positive results.[27]
We also knew of the case of Hector Severino in the Dominican
Republic who had tested positive after a motorbike accident, had been
refused surgery and his wife's fear of his diagnosis had led to her

suicide. Subsequently, Severino has tested HIV negative on two occasions. In 1997, he continues in excellent health.[28]

Now it was our turn to read of Londoner, Tony (he wishes not to reveal his real name). In 1986, at the age of 52, he was diagnosed HIV positive after a routine health check and for six years he thought he had AIDS. 'I was given a death sentence on the strength of one blood test,' he said. His family abandoned him and people refused to even eat with him before checking with their doctors that it was safe. 'I was treated like a leper, like a fiend. When I had dental treatment the dentist wore a helmet and a visor.' He became so afraid he might infect others that he would wash his hands over and over again with bleach until they were raw.[29] Tony was tested again in 1991 and was found to be negative. He asked for his original sample to be retested and that also proved negative. The laboratory concerned was at University College London (UCL), Medical School's Department of Virology, headed by Professor Richard Tedder. Tony decided to take legal action. His solicitor, Alan Bruce of Lloyd & Company has said that Camden and Islington Area Health Authority were not disputing liability and negotiation for a settlement was underway.[30]

We were reminded also of the mystery surrounding the fact that HIV positive children with haemophilia had tested positive for HIV even after their Factor VIII transfusions had been checked and double checked and found to be HIV negative. With sexual transmission out of the question, how could these children possibly have contracted HIV? A faulty batch of Factor VIII must have slipped through, says the orthodoxy. But if this were to be the cause, why did all the other children who received the same batch not become HIV positive?[31]

Our research on the puzzling issue of false positives led us to Rome University where Professor Vittorio Colizzi has discovered that when patients with a blood disorder called thalassaemia were transfused (with HIV antibody negative blood), the more transfusions they received, the more of them tested positive for HIV. That is, they tested positive for antibodies to the primary proteins said to be specific to HIV – p24, gp120 and p41. Colizzi also studied a group of women in Sicily. He chose this region because he wanted to find women who had had sexual intercourse over many years with only one partner. He found that women who had had several children by the same father had, over the years, built up antibodies that produced an HIV positive test result.[32]

We wanted to highlight the issue of false positives – a problem acknowledged by the orthodoxy – but, more importantly, we wanted to go a step further and, through Eleopulos's work, explain that a false positive was a misnomer, that what in fact was being tested for did not exist. Clearly another documentary television programme was beckoning and the ever patient David Lloyd at Channel 4 once again was supportive with some development funds. Working together with Huw Christie, editor of *Continuum* magazine, we selected a group of HIV positive volunteers who were willing to be re-tested for our research project. We devised our own series of preliminary tests to investigate the reliability of the HIV test. Given the death sentence attached to an HIV positive diagnosis and the concomitant fear and discrimination, this was a project that would require very careful handling indeed.

To achieve absolute objectivity, we asked Dr Andrew Taylor at the Robens Institute, at Surrey University, an analytical laboratory well known for its public health concerns, to coordinate our sample testing. He chose a reference laboratory to perform the ELISA HIV test but at this stage he did not reveal the laboratory's identity. Our samples were to be tested on three different test kits. There are more than 20 commercial ELISA HIV test kits on the market. We chose three well known ones from the manufacturers, Murex (who took over the Wellcome's Wellcozyme test), Organon and Pasteur.

Now to select our blood samples. We already knew that people with inflammatory (autoimmune) diseases like rheumatoid arthritis and lupus, but no AIDS symptoms, could test positive. Antibodies generated by TB, candidiasis and malaria could also cross-react with the HIV test; so could the blood of intravenous drug users and alcoholics with hepatitis B. According to Eleopulos, these conditions can produce a very high gammaglobulin (protein) count which can show positive on the ELISA test. We eventually selected a set of 39 blood samples from all over the world to include the above conditions. Our TB samples were flown from Cape Town and our lupus and malaria samples were provided by UCL Medical School.

We then gathered our HIV positive volunteers together. We wanted to test them again through our controlled study on the three different test kits and also at several HIV testing clinics at central London teaching hospitals. There were five diagnosed positive volunteers and one, Peter Nicholls, who thought he was positive because of his risk behaviour. A doctor took blood samples from all six and they were sent off to the Robens Institute. There, Dr Taylor gave them code numbers for a preliminary run and then, to blind the study even further, gave a second batch of the same blood samples a new number for a second run.

By the time our first set of results came back to us, we knew that our samples had been sent to the reference laboratory at UCL's Medical School, under Professor Richard Tedder. Our testing was coordinated there by Stephen Rice. We were surprised to receive the results on both runs from only two test kits, Murex and Organon. At first sight, there was nothing particularly surprising about these results. The diagnosed positives (and Peter Nicholl's sample which we expected to be positive) were all conspicuously positive (over 2.00 optical density) when compared with the other samples which were all negative (in the region of 0.04 optical density). As for the third set of results from the Pasteur test kit, apparently the laboratory had not been satisfied with the 'quality control' on it, but nonetheless agreed to send the results through by fax. Here, indeed, was a very different picture – 19 of the results, including patients with malaria, TB and lupus were in the indeterminate range. That is, they were way above the relative levels detected on the first two test kits and some were verging on positive. According to reference laboratory guidelines, these would have had to be retested.

We then contacted UCL about the Pasteur results and were told that after further checks they were completely satisfied with all three sets of results. Here was a clear example of a significant difference in results between the test kits. At this stage we were not surprised to see that Peter Nicholls had tested positive on all three kits. But later his results were to provide the strongest evidence of the unreliability of the whole testing procedure.

Because Eleopulos had stressed that we should find some samples that were high in gammaglobulin counts (IGG and IGM) we asked a teaching hospital's protein reference laboratory to provide us with some samples from patients who had autoimmune conditions (like rheumatoid arthritis or lupus) but not AIDS defining diseases. We sent four of them to be tested at a central London private testing laboratory. Two days later we received the news that one of them (with the highest gammaglobulin count) had definitely tested positive. No second test was required. Here was a clear example of a patient with an autoimmune disorder that was nothing to do with 'AIDS', testing positive for HIV. How many more of these were there, we wondered?

Now for the second part of our plan. We knew that when information is known (usually through the physician's request form) about an individual's risk factors, for example if he is homosexual or a drug user, an indeterminate result can be interpreted as positive when the individual's clinical notes are taken into consideration. So, to rule out any possible bias we decided to take the diagnosed positives (5) and Peter Nicholls to be tested again at either private clinics or NHS HIV clinics. These six volunteers were gay, but said they were heterosexual at the clinics. The five previously positive volunteers tested consistently positive, but to our astonishment, Peter Nicholls who had been found positive anonymously at UCL six times over (bearing in mind the double run on each of the three test kits) tested negative at two leading London teaching hospitals, St Mary's, Paddington and the Royal Free Hospital. These second tests were performed only a month after the first ones. So, in one month, Nicholls had gone from HIV positive three times to HIV negative twice.

These tests, funded on a shoestring by a television channel and conducted by a small independent production company, should have been performed long ago and on a much larger scale. They show how the HIV test is neither specific nor can it be reproduced satisfactorily. They show that many of our 18,000 diagnosed HIV positive individuals in the UK are bound to be false positives. They also remind us of all the tragic suicides that have taken place after a positive diagnosis with its accompanying and terrifying death sentence. The situation is further aggravated by the recent introduction of home HIV testing kits in the USA. The tests involve pricking your finger with an enclosed lancet, squeezing three drops of blood on to a designated number-coded test card and then mailing the card back to the company for analysis. Seven days later results can be given to you over the telephone. There has been a great deal of controversy about the tests going without any clinical face-to-face counselling, so the manufacturers have opened a free-phone counselling service.

Already, in the USA people are suing the health authorities for 'wrong diagnoses'. A group of lawyers in Miami, Florida and Fort Worth, Texas have 80 pending cases. They predict there will be an avalanche of litigation in the near future. In Miami, lawyer Steve Mitchell took the first case of wrongful diagnosis through the courts in 1993. The case he won involved a woman aged 49 who had not been sexually active for three decades because she had been gang raped in her twenties. She was in hospital for thyroid problems and was offered a free HIV test. She tested positive.

She was told that her positive diagnosis could have resulted from a blood transfusion she had had long ago and that there was no need for a retest. Mitchell's client was put on a drug similar to AZT called ddI. She was ostracized by her community and driven from her church. Her mother washed all her dishes in raw bleach, would not use the same toilet and if her daughter cut herself, bleach would be poured on her open wound. The woman became so distressed, she had to give up custody of her teenage boy and moved to Georgia where she decided to commit suicide. All this time her physical health was good and her T-cell count was 'sky rocketing' (which means very good). Her cousin who was a nurse insisted she be retested. The woman was retested and found negative. She did not believe it. So she was tested twice more and found negative. She believed it – and decided to take legal action. She won and was awarded $600,000 in compensation.

How many more people have, or will in the future, suffer the indescribable horror of being given a 'wrong' ten-year AIDS death sentence? And there are stranger things yet. Clare Thompson in her *Sunday Times Magazine* article did some valuable research into anomalies surrounding being HIV positive.[33] One Los Angeles youngster who was HIV positive at birth had lost HIV at the age of five. The researchers at UCLA AIDS Institute said the virus had been eradicated from the boy's body but was still growing in laboratory test tubes. In Seattle, Judy was found HIV positive at the age of 19 and continued to test positive on three occasions in the next five years. In 1989, she gave birth to a son who was also HIV positive. Yet, in 1992, her second child was born negative while Judy remained positive. Then Judy tested negative.

In 1988, Alfred Saah, a researcher at Johns Hopkins, Baltimore found several of his patients had gone from positive to negative – Fran Peavey from California, for example, who had three positive tests in 1988 and is negative in 1992. Says Saah, 'I was ignored. They said the initial tests must have been contaminated. But I went back and tested again and I was right. I felt like John the Baptist calling in the wilderness. At least I am now back in the fold.' Bill Paxton, a Scottish immunologist working in New York, has found that several high risk but uninfected people had blood cells that could not be infected with HIV, no matter how many doses of virus was added to their blood.

Eric Fuchs, for example, a 39-year-old management consultant in New York, had every reason to believe he should be HIV positive. Although now monogamous, he readily admits to years of promiscuity on the gay scene during the 1970s and 1980s. However, repeated attempts have been made to infect his blood *in vitro* with HIV but without success. He is declared immune to AIDS. Sarah Rowland-Jones at Oxford is investigating several samples of blood that also appear to be immune to AIDS. For example, the wife of a haemophiliac who has remained uninfected although she had unprotected sex with her HIV positive husband for two years before he realized he 'had the disease'.[34]

Positively False: Wrong Tests and Long-Term Survivors

In a further stage of research for Channel 4 we discovered that in Scotland a positive HIV diagnosis requires ELISA tests (the optical density test that measures antibody levels) to be confirmed with a Western blot test (the test that separates into bands each protein/antibody reaction). In England, Philip Mortimer at PHLS recommended a sequence of ELISAs without a Western blot.[35]

We devised a further set of tests, gathering together 16 samples, and sent them to be tested on ELISA in England and on Western blot in Scotland. Four samples that we knew had previously tested positive were included in the 16. These four tested consistently positive in England and Scotland. One of our samples tested negative in England and soundly positive in Scotland. A further five samples tested negative in London and equivocal in Scotland (this meant that one or two of the HIV specific proteins were present). And two samples tested negative in London but with a 'non specific band' in Scotland. This meant that antibodies to proteins close to the HIV specific proteins were present in the Scottish results. These samples were declared neither negative nor positive.

Of our total of 16 samples, 12 were declared negative in London. Of these 12, six or 50 per cent were either positive (1) or equivocal (5) on a Western blot in Scotland. This small set of tests confirmed the published literature on the existence of false positives, but it also shed light on how the interpretation of a test result depends not on a straight positive or negative, but on an assessment of high or low antibody reactions.

If we look at our full sequence of 42 samples (the earlier run of 26 that went through three different test kits and the further 16), we find that two of the 42 had completely contradictory results – either negative then positive or positive then negative – and one tested 'false positive' (when the patient concerned had no AIDS defining diseases or HIV risk). Without even including the equivocal results, we are left with three 'wrong diagnoses'. The Department of Health accepts only a 0.01 per cent degree of inaccuracy in HIV testing, and that even that percentage will be rooted out through further testing. But our small sample found a 7 per cent degree of inaccuracy. This could mean that 1260 of the 18,000 individuals diagnosed HIV positive in the UK are living under a mistaken death sentence. These estimates are conservative, using the orthodoxy's own methods and criteria. However, it is the view of Eleopulos and her colleagues that the whole concept of HIV testing is mistaken because it is based on the indirect identification of something that has not been isolated and cannot provide a gold standard to test against.

Another aspect of our research involved placing advertisements in several gay newspapers and magazines asking for HIV 'long-term survivors' to contact us. We were able to gather together what we described as a 'football' team of long-term survivors. Many of them have been HIV positive for 11 years. One of them had been found positive at a London teaching hospital in the summer of 1996 and then negative two weeks later. The one thing the long-term survivors had in common was that they had refused to take AZT from the very beginning. Several of them said they had seen friends die who went on to AZT and continued with their drug taking habits. Clearly, none of the established principles about HIV and AIDS have stood up to the test. There has been no heterosexual pandemic; AIDS has remained firmly locked into the high-risk groups and AIDS has not behaved like a sexually-transmitted disease should.

It has been ten years since we set out on this journey into the controversy surrounding AIDS. At first we thought the information we were highlighting, through the leading AIDS dissident scientists, would change the world, but the orthodoxy's ranks have remained serried. Considering the mental torment created by an HIV diagnosis, the physical damage caused by AZT, the 100,000 scientific papers about HIV and AIDS that have yet to find the answers about AIDS or to save a single life, these questions remain. How long does it take to shift an entrenched orthodoxy into looking into and funding new avenues of research? Will it take 350 years – the time it took the Catholic Church to absolve Galileo of heresy? Will it take 30 years – the time it took Dr Goldberger to convince his colleagues that pellagra was not infectious but a disease caused by malnutrition? Or will the latest information about the unreliability of the HIV test with the threat of a flood of litigation ahead finally tip the balance? It is a truism that money always speaks. But in the same way that the issue surrounding SMON in Japan was only finally settled in the courts, the impending litigation surrounding AZT damage and wrong diagnoses will change the face of AIDS science forever.

Protease Inhibitors: Another AIDS 'Cure' Fails

As we worked on the research surrounding the HIV test, we were also plunged into the current controversy surrounding the new drug cocktail for AIDS involving protease inhibitor drugs (PIs) and the tests used to check whether the drugs have succeeded in reducing an individual's 'viral load'.

A further brief period of development was granted us by David Lloyd at Channel 4, and Mark Galloway, the editor of Channel 4's *Health Alert* series, has also expressed interest in aspects of our HIV test investigations.

A certain euphoria has surrounded the introduction of the new and enormously expensive triple therapy cocktail for AIDS. There have been stories of a 'Lazarus effect' with patients suddenly springing back to life and hospital wards emptying out. But, for some the effects have been short-lived. David Roemer, for example, was on the front page of the *New York Times* when he was able to take up his bed and take on his job again. Two months later he was back on the front page – dead.[36]

The honeymoon period is now over and doubts about the wisdom of prescribing this cocktail to people with AIDS and to people who have tested HIV positive with no symptons of AIDS have begun to creep in. PIs were licensed in the USA through a fast track procedure after the trials were prematurely terminated. They can have serious adverse effects, there is no scientific proof that they work and the manufacturers themselves say the drugs cannot cure AIDS. However, the clamour for treatment from some AIDS pressure groups has led to a frenzy of speculation as to how they should be funded and at the expense of what existing care and treatment facilities.

The new cocktail involves two drugs (one of them AZT or an analogue) that allegedly prevent HIV from integrating into a cell, and another, a protease inhibitor (PI), which is said to block the HIV protease enzyme, thereby preventing the packaging and releasing of newly-made viruses into the bloodstream.

The three main protease inhibitors on the market are:

indinavir	Crixivan	Merck, Sharp & Dohme
ritanovir	Norvir	Abbott Laboratories
saquinavir	Invirase	Roche

PIs were licensed after a US$ 5 million federal research study conducted by the US National Institute of Allergy and Infectious Diseases

(NIAID) involving 1156 AIDS patients. The study, at 19 US medical centres, was halted in midstream in February 1997 because the trialists declared that results, thus far, were so good that it would be unethical to prevent patients from benefiting from the new drug combination (estimated cost $15,000 a year). It was announced that the number of deaths and AIDS related illnesses in the group taking triple therapy were almost half those of the group taking two drugs.

The researchers said that for technical reasons it could not be said that the difference in deaths was statistically significant. Nonetheless, the study leader, Dr Scott Hammer, said enigmatically, 'It is fair to say there was a reduction in mortality that is consistent with the overall results.' Dr Anthony Fauci, director of NIAID, said that combination treatments that included protease inhibitors '*can* reduce risk of death' (emphasis added).[37] These were the trials that led to the licensing of PIs.

Many doctors are ambivalent about the current euphoria that surrounds PIs. Professor Brian Gazzard at a lecture on the triple therapy cocktail at the Royal College of Physicians in November 1997 was cautious about the more aggressive American approach to treatment. Gazzard's tone reflected a creeping disillusion surrounding PIs and, for that matter, any real advances in AIDS therapy. He acknowledged that AZT monotherapy had failed and concluded with the surprising remark that perhaps everything he had said that evening was wrong. Maybe 10 per cent was right but which 10 per cent remained to be seen, he said. Dr Donald Abrams, director of the AIDS programme at San Francisco General Hospital, does not describe himself as a cheerleader for antiviral therapy. At a medical school seminar he said, 'I have a large population of people who have chosen not to take any antivirals. ... They've watched their friends go on the antiviral bandwagon and die, so they've chosen to remain naive [not to take antivirals].'[38]

The 1987 data sheet information in the UK about saquinavir (Invirase) from Roche says: 'Patients should be informed that saquinavir is not a cure for HIV infection and that they may continue to acquire illnesses associated with advanced HIV infection, including opportunistic infections.'

The US equivalent, Physicians' Desk Reference, has a warning that is not included in the UK information. 'WARNING – The indication for Invirase for the treatment of HIV infection is based on changes in surrogate markers. At present there are no results from controlled clinical trials evaluating the effect of regimens containing Invirase on survival or the clinical progression of HIV infection, such as the occurrences of opportunistic infections or malignancies.'[39]

Toxicity

Dr David Raznick, research scientist at the University of California, Berkeley, who spent 20 years developing PIs for other conditions, describes how the toxicity associated with PIs means that the liver is blocked from processing the drug's own toxicities. The toxins build up in the liver and then the 'crash' can be very sudden.

Toxic effects are a major problem. Hepatic and renal impairment are listed as well as diarrhoea, headaches, peripheral neuropathy and rare associated cases of severe skin problems, acute myeloblastic leukaemia, jaundice, polyarthritis and pancreatitis leading to death.

'Crix belly' is another side effect. Crixivan and other PIs affect the digestive system and individuals have suffered massive swelling of the stomach associated with decreased digestion.

A recent study from San Francisco General Hospital shows that the drug failed in 53 per cent of people taking it. It is currently held that between 35 and 50 per cent cannot tolerate the adverse effects.[40] Another study from San Francisco revealed an increased risk of the AIDS defining condition – cytomegalovirus retinitis – in people taking PIs.[41]

On 11 June 1997 the US Food and Drug Administration issued a warning to doctors saying that thousands of patients taking protease inhibitors should be closely watched for an unexpected side effect – diabetes. Although the warning said that the estimated 100,000 Americans taking the drug should not stop because the diabetes risk appeared to be small, they were concerned about 83 patients who had contracted diabetes or had their existing diabetes suddenly worsen after they began taking PIs.

Information about PIs from several London AIDS drop-in centres has been conflicting. At one we heard the new combination therapy had helped one man put on weight, while another said he could not handle the regimen involving 20 tablets a day taken an hour after meals with no food for three hours after that. At another centre, we were informed that over the previous ten days three men taking triple therapy had died.

In October last year, 31-year-old Philip Kay died after taking two and a half tablets of Ecstacy (MDMA). He was also on the PI ritanovir (Norvir). Abbott UK, the manufacturers of Norvir admitted that, because PIs affect the liver's ability to process other drugs, the level of Ecstasy in Philip's blood could have increased threefold. The coroner, however, concluded that there had been a fatal tenfold increase in Philip's levels of Ecstasy.[42]

The Cost

The American approach is to give the drugs early to people with no symptoms of AIDS. But in the UK some specialists are more cautious. Professor Ian Weller (who conducted the AZT Concorde trials) says, 'I am uncomfortable about the emphasis on early intervention when we really don't know that that's the right thing to do. ... Without any drugs, 50 per cent of people will be still perfectly well ten years after they become infected. We may not have the right drugs to commit people to many years of therapy.'[43]

If the American approach were to be adopted in the UK it would mean that the 18,000 diagnosed positive individuals in the UK would be under 'ferocious pressure' to go on the very costly triple therapy. Triple therapy costs £15,000 per year per patient (£10,000 for the drugs and approximately £5000 for the viral load tests that are used to assess the effects of the drug cocktails. The total budget for AIDS (including treatment care, community support and research) in the UK for 1997/8 was £260 million, almost exactly what the total triple therapy costs would be.

The Inner London HIV Health Commissioner's Group has announced that seven area health authorities will be making drastic reductions in money spent on areas such as advice centres, buddying/befriending,

pastoral care and drop-in centres, complementary or alternative therapies, as well as reducing the number of hospice beds, in order to
finance the new drug cocktails.

Another concern involves the fear that health authorities will be
sued if they do not provide triple therapy. Dr Raymond Brettle at City
Hospital in Edinburgh is worried about the costs involved in PI
therapy. He has already seen services in his hospital cut when only
dual therapy had to be paid for. He feels triple therapy will have
drastic effects on other services. However, if PIs are not funded, he
foresees a repetition of the precedent set in a case involving North
Derby Area Health Authority, when a patient with multiple sclerosis
was not given beta-interferon. She sued and won her case on the
grounds that the authority was obliged to provide therapy if there was
evidence that it was effective. This fear of litigation among health
authorities is forcing them into increasing their drugs budgets at the
expense of other care facilities.

Most of the Western world believes that PIs are saving the lives of
people with AIDS. But is this right? In 1996, in New York City with 16
per cent of US AIDS diagnoses, AIDS deaths dropped by 30 per cent.
Health officials did not attribute the drop to protease inhibitors.
According to May Ann Chiasson, assistant health commissioner for
New York City, the AIDS death rate began to fall *before the main drugs
were introduced*. She suggested the decline may be linked more closely
to better general health practices and more effective treatment of
opportunistic infections.

AIDS drug therapy has reached a stage whereby pressure from the
consumer (people with AIDS) has pushed the drug manufacturers into
'fast tracking' drugs that have not been through the normal clinical
test procedures before being licensed. What is the justification for this
rush to judgement? How long will it take before PIs are considered to
be a failure?

Simon Collins, writing in *Positive Nation*, says that for people who
are currently well, the decision as to whether or not to start therapy is
a worrying one. 'You have to understand the role as a guinea pig. Your
doctor will be unable to answer the most important questions you ask.
How long will this extend my life? What are the long-term dangers?'[44]

And John Stevens writes: 'We live in extraordinary times. Never before have so many combinations of pharmaceuticals been taken for such extended periods of time; drug "cocktails" that bring benefits as well as substantial long-term side effects, known or otherwise.'[45]

We live in extraordinary times indeed. Exactly ten years ago trials for AZT were prematurely terminated and the drug was rushed onto the market. Now, AZT on its own is considered by the AIDS establishment to have failed. And yet it is still included in some of the new cocktails. But then experience shows that it can take ten years for ineffective and dangerous drugs to be withdrawn from the market.

It has been a decade since we started to investigate the controversy about AIDS. After the £2000 million spent in the UK on AIDS and the $40,000 million spent in the USA, none of the established principles about HIV and AIDS have stood up to the test. There has been no heterosexual pandemic; AIDS has remained firmly locked into the high risk groups; AIDS has not behaved like a sexually transmitted disease should and no cure for AIDS has been found.

Appendix A

Summary of SCAM Document Submitted to MRC with Objections to the PENTA Trial Protocol

Medical Research Council, PENTA 1 Trial,
3 February 1992 (Amended 12 August 1992)

1. *The design of the study was fundamentally flawed. The age range for the study was 18 months to 16 years. This implied that a child could live to the age of 16 with HIV and remain healthy. (Remember only children who had not presented with symptoms of AIDS qualified for entry into the study.) Given the toxic effects of AZT, there was no chance that a healthy 18-month-old HIV positive child would remain healthy or even survive for 14 years on high doses of AZT.*

2. *The trial recommended that when a child, whether on placebo or on the drug, 'fails to thrive' and 'definitely needs AZT', it should automatically be given AZT (open label transfer). As the effects of AZT are often indistinguishable from the symptoms of AIDS itself it would not be possible to know whether a child was genuinely failing to thrive, or suffering from the effects of AZT. If the latter, it could be lethal to keep them on the drug.*

3. *The recommended dosage of AZT for both adults and children worried our advisers. They pointed out that the statutory information supplied by Wellcome to the US Physicians' Desk Reference (PDR) regarding toxicity thresholds for safe doses of AZT was wrong. This information had never been amended since the first entries were made by Wellcome in the PDR in 1988. However, since then, five separate studies (see Chapter 11, note 26) had shown that AZT is 1000 times more toxic to healthy cells than is claimed. In the PDR the threshold for AZT's toxicity to lymphocytes was set at 20 micromoles, which is equal to a 500 mg dose per day in an adult. Yet the PENTA trial's doses in children (600 mg/m2/day) were equal to a dose of 1080 mg per day in an adult. In terms of molar concentrations in the body, this was equal to 43 micromoles. Therefore, according to the five independent studies quoted above, the AZT concentrations of the PENTA trial were up to 43 times more toxic to the cell than was tolerable and therefore cytopathic (cell killing).*

4. *The PENTA trial letter to parents said 'We know from studies in adults that AZT helps people who are ill with AIDS making them feel better and allowing them to live longer.' This was a false claim as there is no scientific evidence to prove that AZT makes people 'feel better'. And the statement about living longer was based on the phase II trials, which we have already demonstrated were flawed.*

5. *The parents' letter also stated that AZT could cause a drop in white blood cells leading to anaemia, but that this was 'reversible if AZT is stopped or the dose is reduced'. This was not always true as Mir and Costello had reported in their letter to the* Lancet *(11 November 1988,*

pp. 1195–6). No mention was made in the letter of the known carcinogenic potential of AZT *(Medical Research Council,* Handbook, *1992, p. 3).*

6. *It has been standard practice for at least 40 years to conduct radio-labelled metabolism studies on any new drug to see where the drug is absorbed in the body. A thorough literature search has shown that this had not been done with* AZT. *It is hard to conceive of any reason why this is so, and our advisers feared that the results of such work would demonstrate that* AZT *is metabolized mainly in the intestines and bone marrow, and not at all in T-cells (as was alleged.)*

Notes

Preface

1. Interview for *Reappraising AIDS*, Group for the scientific reappraisal of HIV and AIDS, 1994.
2. Peter Deusberg, 'Foreword' to Jad Adams's, *AIDS: The HIV Myth*, Macmillan, London, 1989.
3. David J. Miller and Michael Hersen (eds) *Research Fraud in the Behavioural and Biomedical Sciences*, John Wiley, New York/Chichester, 1992, p. 251 (ISBN 0–471–52068–3). Taken from review of the book by John Lauritsen, *Lancet*, 8 August 1992.
4. Peter Duesberg, 'Retroviruses as carcinogens and pathogens: expectations and reality', *Cancer Research*, vol. 47, no. 5 CNREA 8, 1 March 1987, pp. 1199–220.
5. Peter Duesberg, 'AIDS epidemiology: inconsistencies with human immunodeficiency virus and with infectious disease', *PNAS*, vol. 88, February 1991, pp. 1575–9.
6. Kary Mullis to Neville Hodgkinson, *Sunday Times* science correspondent, 26 April 1992.
7. Christopher Dunkley, *Financial Times*, 1 December 1993.
8. Wembley Stadium speech, London, 20 April 1992.
9. Andrew Scott, *Pirates of the Cell*, Basil Blackwell, London, revised 1987 (ISBN 0–631–15637–2).
10. Eleni Eleopulos et al., 'The isolation of HIV: has it really been achieved? The case against', *Continuum*, vol. 4, no. 3, September/October 1996; Eleni Eleopulos et al., 'Why no whole virus?', *Continuum*, vol. 4, no. 5, February/March 1997.
11. Bryan J. Ellison and P. H. Duesberg, *Why We Will Never Win the War on AIDS*, Inside Story Communications, El Cerrito, California, 1994.
12. Ibid.
13. Soda, T. (ed.) 'Drug-induced sufferings: medical, pharmaceutical, and legal aspects', *Excerpta medica*, Amsterdam, 1980.

Chapter 1: Journey into Dissidence

1. 'The pill generation', *Dispatches*, Channel 4, 18 May 1994.
2. 'The cot death poisonings', *The Cook Report* (2 programmes), Central TV, 17 November and 1 December 1994.

Chapter 2: AIDS: The Unheard Voices

1. Peter Duesberg, (letter) *Science*, vol. 257, 1848, 25 September 1992.
2. Wei and Ho, *Nature*, vol. 373, 1995, p. 117; David Ho, *Nature*, vol. 373, p. 123.
3. Peter Duesberg and Harvey Bialy, letter to *Nature*, 18 May 1995.
4. Mark Craddock, 'HIV: Science by press conference', in P. H. Duesberg, *Aids: Virus or Drug Induced?*, Kluwer Academic Publishers, Netherlands, 1996, pp. 127–30; Serge Lang, *Challenges*, Springer Verlag, New York, November 1997.
5. *AIDS: The Unheard Voices*, *Dispatches*, Channel 4, programme transcript, 1987.
6. Ibid.
7. Ibid.
8. Ibid.
9. Ibid.
10. Ibid.
11. Ibid.
12. Liz Cowley, *Daily Mail*, 13 November, 1987.
13. Christopher Tookey, *Sunday Telegraph*, 15 November 1987.
14. *Lancet*, 6 May 1989, p. 1031.
15. Beverly Griffin, 'Burden of Proof', *Nature*, vol. 338, 20 April 1989, p. 670.
16. Duncan Campbell, 'AIDS: The Duesberg Myth', *New Scientist*, 6 May 1989, pp. 60–1.
17. Martin Walker, *Dirty Medicine*, Slingshot Publications, London, 1993, pp. 370–6. (Duncan Campbell speaking at London School of Economics, 13 April 1989.)
18. Ibid.
19. Ibid.
20. *New Scientist*, 3 June 1989, p. 71.
21. Anthony Pinching, 'A Flat Earth Society Manifesto', *Independent*, 17 April 1989.
22. John Stuart Mill, *Liberty*, Chapter 2.

Chapter 3: Life in Backrooms and Bathhouses

1. 'The AIDS catch', *Dispatches*, Channel 4, programme transcript 1992.
2. Michael Callen, *Surviving AIDS*, Harper & Row, London, September 1990.
3. Michael Callen and Richard Berkowitz, 'We know who we are', *New York Native*, 8–21 November 1982.
4. 'The AIDS catch', *Dispatches*, Channel 4, rushes transcript, 1992.
5. Ibid.
6. Ibid.
7. Dennis Altman, *Homosexual Oppression and Liberation*, Plymbridge, Boston, 1993.
8. David Black, 'The plague years', *Rolling Stone*, no. 444, 28 March 1985.
9. 'The AIDS catch', *Dispatches*, Channel 4, programme transcript 1990.
10. John Lauritsen, *The AIDS War*, Asklepios, New York, 1993, p. 192 (ISBN 0–943742–08–0).
11. Larry Kramer, *Faggots*, Minerva, New York, 1990.
12. John Lauritsen, *The AIDS War*, op. cit. p. 426.

13. Ian Peacock, 'Pop till you drop!', *Boyz Magazine*, 16 October 1993.
14. Cass Mann, St Stephens Hospital workshop, September 1987.
15. Camille Paglia, *Sex, Art, and American Culture*, Viking, London, 1992.
16. David Black, *Rolling Stone*, no. 444, 28 March 1985.
17. Peter Duesberg, 'The role of drugs in the origin of AIDS', *Biomed & Pharmacother*, vol. 46, 1992, Elsevier, Paris, pp. 3–15.
18. Maurizio Lucà Moretti, *JIMHA*, vol. 1, no. 1, January–April 1992.
19. Jad Adams, *AIDS: The HIV Myth*, Macmillan, London, 1989.
20. David Black, *Rolling Stone*, no. 444, 28 March 1985.
21. 'Amsterdam Alternative AIDS Conference' Meditel Productions, rushes transcript, 1992.

Chapter 4: Hunting the Human Retrovirus

1. *Science*, 12 November 1993, p. 981.
2. Peter Duesberg, 'Retroviruses as carcinogens and pathogens: expectations and reality', *Cancer Research*, vol. 47, no. 5, CNREA 8, 1 March 1987, pp. 1199–220.
3. Robert Gallo, Introduction for P. H. Duesberg, Neth, Gallo, Greaves and Janka (eds), 'Modern Trends in Human Leukemia VI', *Haematology and Blood Transfusion*, vol. 29, Springer-Verlag, Berlin and Heidelberg, 1985.
4. *New Scientist*, 3 March 1988.
5. Anthony Liversidge, *Spin Magazine*, February 1988.
6. Ibid.
7. 'The AIDS catch', *Dispatches*, Channel 4, programme transcript, 1990.
8. *Reappraising AIDS*, recorded interview series, 1994.
9. Robert Gallo, *Virus Hunting, AIDS Cancer and the Human Retrovirus*, Harper Collins, New York, 1991.
10. Peter Duesberg, 'On Virus Hunting' *New York Native*, 29 April 1991.
11. Barry Werth, 'The AIDS windfall', *New England Monthly*, June 1988.
12. Stephen S. Hall, 'Gadfly in the Ointment', *Hippocrates*, September/October 1988.
13. Peter Duesberg, 'Oncogenes and Cancer', letter, *Science*, vol. 267, 1995, p. 1407.
14. Robert Gallo, *Virus Hunting,* op. cit.
15. Abraham Karpas letter to Serge Lang, February 1993, in Bryan J. Ellison and P. H. Duesberg, *Why We Will Never Win the War on AIDS*, Inside Story Communications, El Cerrito, California, 1994.
16. Jad Adams, *AIDS: The HIV Myth*, Macmillan, London, 1989, p. 43.
17. Robert Gallo, *Virus Hunting*, op. cit.
18. *AIDS: The Unheard Voices*, *Dispatches*, Channel 4, rushes transcript, 1987.
19. Robert Gallo, *Virus Hunting*, op. cit.
20. Robert Gallo, letter to Carlo Croce, 10 February 1986.
21. William Heseltine, letter to Robert Gallo, 24 February 1986.
22. Robert Gallo, *Virus Hunting*, op. cit.
23. K. Tajima and T. Kuroishi, *Japan J. Clin. Oncol*, vol. 15, 1985, pp. 423–30.
24. Peter Duesberg, 'Retroviruses as carcinogens and pathogens: expectations and reality', *Cancer Research*, vol. 47, no. 5, CNREA 8, 1 March 1987, pp. 1199–220.

25. Ibid.

26. John Lauritsen, *The AIDS War*, Asklepios, New York, 1993, pp. 50–1 (ISBN 0–943742–08–0).

27. Robert Gallo, *Virus Hunting*, op. cit.

28. Bryan J. Ellison and P. H. Duesberg, *Why We Will Never Win the War on AIDS*, Inside Story Communications, El Cerrito, California, 1994.

29. F. Barre-Sinoussi et al., *Science*, vol. 220, May 1983, pp. 868–71.

30. Personal conversation with Peter Duesberg, 1989.

31. Celia Farber, 'Fatal distraction', *Spin Magazine*, June 1992.

32. Interview in Toledo by Javier Manero Vargas and Miguel Albinana, in Alfredo Embid (ed.) *Repensar el SIDA: lo que no os han dicho*, Madrid, 1994 (ISBN 84–88346–06–9).

33. Barry Werth, 'The AIDS windfall', *New England Monthly*, June 1988.

34. *Omni Magazine* (interview), December 1988.

35. John Crewdson, 'The great AIDS quest: science under the microscope', *Chicago Tribune*, 19 November 1989.

36. Robert Gallo, letter to *Nature*, vol. 351, 30 May 1991, p. 358.

37. Elaine Richman, *The Sciences*, November/December 1996.

38. *Nature*, vol. 326, 2 April 1987.

39. Jad Adams, '*AIDS: The HIV Myth*, op. cit.

40. Ibid.

41. Herb Frazier, *The Post and Courier* (Charleston, South Carolina), 16 March 1995.

42. Elaine Richman, *The Sciences*, November/December 1996.

43. David Perlman, *San Francisco Chronicle*, 14 February 1997.

44. Daniel Greenberg, *Lancet*, vol. 335, 12 May 1990, pp. 1148–9.

45. Personal conversations, 1990

46. John Crewdson, *Chicago Tribune*, 14 April 1991.

47. Barbara J. Culliton, 'Gallo reports mystery break-in', *Science*, vol. 250, 1990, p. 250.

48. Robert Gallo, *Virus Hunting*, op. cit.

49. Robert Gallo, letter to *Nature*, vol. 351, 30 May 1991, p. 358.

50. Robert Gallo, *Virus Hunting*, op. cit.

Chapter 5: Plague Terror

1. *Sunday Telegraph*, 18 June 1995.

2. *New York Times*, 15 June 1995.

3. *Sunday Times*, 2 November 1986.

4. Ibid.

5. John Lauritsen, 'Latex Lunacy', *New York Native*, 4 July 1988.

6. *Hot 'n Healthy Times*, Eroticus Publications, 1150 Bryant Street, San Francisco, CA 94103, 1986.

7. Ibid.

8. *The Works: Drugs Sex and AIDS*, San Francisco AIDS Foundation, 25 May 1987.

9. *New England Journal of Medicine*, *NEJM*, 1989, vol. 320, p. 1458.

10. *Guardian*, 1 December 1989.
11. *Guardian*, 27 June 1990.
12. *Guardian*, 1 December 1989.
13. *Independent*, 14 January 1988.
14. *Guardian*, 12 June 1989.
15. *Guardian*, 15 February 1989; *OPCS Monitor*, PP2 89/1, HMSO, London.
16. *Lancet*, 5 November 1988.
17. *Sunday Tribune*, Oakland, 21 May 1989.
18. *Daily Telegraph*, 20 June 1988.
19. *The Times*, 4 January 1990.
20. *Guardian*, 13 January 1989.
21. *Sun*, 24 January 1990.
22. Donation from Gareth James, Director, HEAL London Trust.
23. Bryan J. Ellison and P. H. Duesberg, *Why We Will Never Win the War on AIDS*, Inside Story Communications, El Cerrito, California, 1994.
24. Ibid.
25. Ibid.
26. Ibid.
27. *OPCS Monitor*, PP2 89/1, HMSO, London.
28. David Mellor, personal conversation, 1994.
29. *Lancet*, vol. 341, 3 April 1993.
30. Ibid.; Gordon Stewart, 'AIDS and the ethics of programmed compassion', *Bulletin of Medical Ethics*, March 1995.
31. Gordon Stewart, letter to Meditel, 8 September 1995.
32. Gordon Stewart, letter to Meditel, 4 September 1995.
33. James Le Fanu, *Sunday Telegraph*, 4 December 1988.
34. James Le Fanu, *Sunday Telegraph*, 21 July 1991; *The Times*, 11 February 1992.
35. Victoria Macdonald, 'Who are they getting at?', *Sunday Telegraph*, 19 November 1989.

Chapter 6: The AIDS Catch

1. Peter Duesberg, 'HIV and AIDS: correlation but not causation', *PNAS*, vol. 86, pp. 755–64.
2. *Sunday Telegraph*, 1 May 1989.
3. *Sunday Telegraph*, 11 June 1989.
4. Letter to Igor Dawid, 14 July 1988, Meditel archive.
5. Peter Duesberg, 'HIV and AIDS: Correlation but not causation', *PNAS*, op. cit.
6. Peter Duesberg, 'AIDS epidemiology: inconsistencies with human immunodeficiency virus and with infectious disease', *PNAS*, vol. 88, pp. 1572–9, February 1991.
7. 'The AIDS catch', *Dispatches*, Channel 4, rushes transcript, 1990.
8. 'The AIDS catch', *Dispatches*, Channel 4, programme transcript, 1990.
9. Callen and Berkowitz, 'We know who we are', *New York Native*, 8–21 November 1982.

10. 'The AIDS catch', *Dispatches*, Channel 4, programme transcript, 1990.
11. Ibid.
12. Ibid.
13. *Lancet*, vol. 335, 21 April 1990.
14. Robert Root-Bernstein, 'Do we know the cause(s) of AIDS?', *Perspectives in Biology and Medicine*, vol. 33, pp. 480–500, 1990.
15. 'The AIDS catch', programme transcript, 1990.
16. 'The AIDS catch', rushes transcript, 1990.
17. J. R. Berger et al., 'Progressive multifocal leukoencephalopathy 30 years later', *Annals of Internal Medicine*, vol. 107, 1987, pp. 78–87.
18. 'The AIDS catch', programme transcript, 1990.
19. 'The AIDS catch', rushes transcript, 1990.
20. Ibid.
21. 'The AIDS catch', programme transcript, 1990.
22. 'The AIDS catch', rushes transcript, 1990.
23. 'The AIDS catch', programme transcript, 1990.

Chapter 7: Fall Out

1. D. A. Rees, letter to Sir George Russell, 19 June 1990.
2. Hilary Curtis, letter to David Lloyd, 18 June 1990.
3. *British Medical Journal*, vol. 300, 16 June 1990.
4. *New Scientist*, 16 June 1990.
5. *Capital Gay*, 22 June 1990.
6. Hal Satterthwaite, British Medical Association, Newsletter no. 1.
7. *Independent*, 22 June 1990.
8. *The Times*, 14 June, 1990.
9. *Financial Times*, 13 June, 1990.
10. *Independent*, 18 June 1990.
11. *Independent*, 20 June 1990.
12. *Independent* on Sunday, 17 June 1990.
13. *Guardian*, 23 June, 1990.
14. *Guardian*, 29 June 1990.
15. *Guardian*, 13 July 1990.
16. *Guardian*, 31 July 1990
17. *Nature*, vol. 345, 21 June 1990, pp. 659–60.
18. Ibid.
19. Ibid.
20. Peter Duesberg, 'Weiss, Jaffe and the germ theory of AIDS', 12 July 1990, Meditel archive.
21. Peter Duesberg, letter to *Nature*, 18 July 1990.
22. *Nature*, vol. 346 , 30 August 1990.
23. Beverly Griffin, 'AIDS/HIV: a necessary factor but not a sufficient explanation?', submission to the *Lancet*, 20 November 1991. Personal communication, 1 May 1992.
24. Joseph Schwartz, *Creative Moment*, Jonathan Cape, London, 1994.

25. Joseph Schwartz, letter to *Nature*, 25 June 1990.
26. *Nature*, vol. 353, 26 September 1991.
27. *Science*, 14 September 1991.
28. *New Scientist*, 21 September 1991.
29. *Nature*, vol. 353, 26 September 1991.
30. M. S. Ascher et al., *Nature*, vol. 362, 1993, pp. 103–4.
31. M. T. Schechter, *Lancet*, 13 March 1993, p. 658.
32. M. S. Ascher et al., *Nature*, op. cit.
33. Peter Duesberg, letter to *Nature*, 15 May 1993.
34. *Nature*, vol. 363, 13 May 1993.
35. Peter Duesberg, telephone conversation, March 1993.
36. *Lancet*, vol. 341, 10 April 1993, p. 957.
37. Peter Duesberg, *Inventing the AIDS Virus*, Regnery Publishing, Inc., Washington DC, 1996; John Cole, letter to Peter Duesberg, 22 October 1990, p. 399.
38. Peter Duesberg, letter to John Cole, 4 January 1991, Meditel archive.
39. Broadcasting Complaints Commission, complaint from the Wellcome Foundation – Adjudication, 23 May 1991.
40. Nick Partridge, Terrence Higgins Trust, letter to the Broadcasting Complaints Commission, 1 October 1990.
41. The Broadcasting Complaints Commission, Complaint from the Terrence Higgins Trust, Frontliners (UK) Ltd and Positively Women – Adjudication, 23 May 1991.
42. Ibid.

Chapter 8: AZT: Cause for Concern

1. Elinor Burkett, *AZT: Cause for Concern*, programme transcript, *Dispatches*, Channel 4, 1992.
2. Ibid.
3. *Lancet*, 19 November 1988.
4. *New York Native*, articles include: 'AZT on trial', 'On the AZT front', 'AZT watch', 'AZT and cancer', 'AZT: iatrogenic genocide' and 'HIV voodoo from Burroughs Wellcome'. Published between 1987 and 1994.
5. Celia Farber, 'Sins of omission: the AZT scandal', *Spin Magazine*, November 1989.
6. Peter Duesberg, 'AIDS epidemiology: inconsistencies with human immunodeficiency virus and with infectious disease.' *PNAS*, USA, vol. 88, February 1991, pp. 1572–9.
7. Peter Duesberg, 'The role of drugs in the origin of AIDS', *Biomed & Pharmacother*, vol. 46, 1992, pp. 3–15.
8. Brian Deer, *Sunday Times*, 16 April 1989 and 30 April 1989.
9. Duncan Campbell, 'The AIDS scam', *New Statesman and Society*, 24 June 1988.
10. Addendum 91 to Medical Officer Review of FDA 19, p. 655.
11. Ibid.
12. Barbara Spitzig, FDA investigator, 'For cause establishment inspection report of Massachusetts General Hospital and Robert Schooley, MD', October and November 1986.

Notes

13. *AZT: Cause for Concern*, *Dispatches* Channel 4, rushes transcript, 1992.
14. Barbara Spitzig, op. cit.
15. 'AZT on trial' conference, London 1993. *Diary of an AIDS Dissident*, Meditel, programme transcript, 1994.
16. John Lauritsen, *The AIDS War*, Asklepios, New York, 1993.
17. Harvey Chernov, Review and Evaluation of Pharmacology and Toxicology Data (AZT), Food and Drug Administration document, NDA 19–655, 2 December 1986, amendments, 16 and 19 December 1986.
18. Ibid.
19. John Lauritsen, 'AZT and Cancer', *New York Native*, 30 October 1989.
20. J. M. Pluda, R. Yarchoan and S. Broder et al., *Annals of Internal Medicine*, vol. 113, no. 4.
21. Ibid.
22. *Positive Benefits: Wellcome's Anti-HIV Agent, Zidovudine*, Wellcome Foundation information booklet, 1992.
23. *AZT: Cause for Concern*, *Dispatches*, Channel 4, programme transcript, 1992.
24. Ibid.
25. P. Volberding et al., 'Zidovudine in asymptomatic human immunodeficiency virus infection', *New England Journal of Medicine*, vol. 322, no. 14, 5 April 1990.
26. *AZT: Cause for Concern*, Channel 4, programme transcript, 1992.
27. *AZT: Cause for Concern*, *Dispatches*, Channel 4, rushes transcript, 1992.
28. Ibid.
29. *AZT: Cause for Concern*, *Dispatches*, Channel 4, programme transcript, 1992.
30. Dr Martin Sherwood, letter to Meditel, 19 November 1991.
31. John D. Hamilton et al., 'A controlled trial of early versus late treatment with zidovudine in symptomatic human immunodeficiency virus infection', Department of Veterans Affairs, *New England Journal of Medicine*, vol. 326, no. 7, 13 February 1992, pp. 437–86.
32. *AZT: Cause for Concern*, *Dispatches*, Channel 4, programme transcript, 1992.
33. Ibid.
34. Dr A. Wu, *Journal of Acquired Immune Deficiency Syndromes*, vol. 3, 1990, pp. 683–90; Dr A. Wu, *Journal of Acquired Immune Deficiency Syndromes*, vol. 6, 1993, pp. 452–8.
35. *AZT: Cause for Concern*, *Dispatches*, Channel 4, rushes transcript, 1992.
36. *UK Data Sheet Compendium*, 1992; *US Physicians Desk Reference*, 1992.
37. *AZT: Cause for Concern*, *Dispatches*, Channel 4, rushes transcript, 1992.
38. P. Volberding et al., 'Zidovudine in asymptomatic human immunodeficiency virus infection', *New England Journal of Medicine*, vol. 322, no. 14, 5 April 1990.
39. *AZT: Cause for Concern*, *Dispatches*, Channel 4, rushes transcript, 1992.
40. *AZT: Cause for Concern*, *Dispatches*, Channel 4, programme transcript, 1992.
41. Ibid.
42. Ibid.
43. *AZT: Cause for Concern*, *Dispatches*, Channel 4, rushes transcript, 1992.
44. Ibid.
45. Ibid.
46. *AZT: Cause for Concern*, *Dispatches*, Channel 4, programme transcript, 1992.

47. Ibid.
48. *USA Today*, 12 November 1991.
49. *Observer*, 24 November 1991.
50. Ibid.
51. The *San Francisco Enquirer*, 8 December 1991.
52. Ibid.
53. *Los Angeles Times*, 3 November 1996.
54. Ibid.
55. Professor Ian Weller, letter to Liz Forgan, 10 February 1992.
56. Dr S. M. Wood, letter to Meditel, 6 March 1992.
57. Professor W. Asscher, letter to Meditel, 2 April 1992.
58. David Concar, 'Patients abandon AIDS drug after TV show', *New Scientist*, 13 July 1991, p. 13.
59. John D. Hamilton, op. cit. 1992.
60. Wellcome, Dear Doctor letter, 3 February 1992.
61. Brian Deer, 'AIDS Doctors Attack Drug Claims', *Sunday Times*, August 1993.
62. *New Scientist*, 7 August 1993.
63. Wellcome, Dear Doctor letter, *Dispatches* Programme, Channel 4 Television, February 1992.
64. Brian Robb, letter to Michael Grade, 24 February 1992.
65. Michael Grade, letter to Brian Robb, 23 March 1992.
66. D. S. Freestone, letter, *Lancet*, vol. 339, 7 March 1992, p. 626.
67. Joan Shenton, letter to the *Lancet*, vol. 339, 28 March 1992, p. 806.
68. Liz Hunt, 'BMA under fire over AIDS film', *Independent on Sunday*, 23 May 1993.
69. Neville Hodgkinson, *Sunday Times*, 30 May 1993.
70. Dr S. J. Mansfield, letter to Dr John Hamilton, 24 February 1992.
71. Dr John Hamilton, letter to Dr S. J. Mansfield, 9 March 1992.

Chapter 9: Amsterdam and All That

1. Robert Root-Bernstein, *Rethinking AIDS*, The Free Press, New York, 1993.
2. *Sunday Times*, 26 April 1992.
3. William Leith, The *Independent on Sunday*, 10 May 1992.
4. *The Times*, 11 May 1992.
5. Ibid.
6. *The Times*, 15 May 1992.
7. Neville Hodgkinson, *Sunday Times*, 17 May 1992.
8. Paul Woolwich, letter to Joan Shenton, 8 May 1992.
9. 'Alternative AIDS Conference', Meditel Productions, transmitted on Sky News, May 1992.
10. Ibid.
11. Ibid.
12. *Nature*, vol. 349, 31 January 1991.
13. *Independent on Sunday*, 20 January 1991.
14. Robin Weiss, letter , *Nature*, vol. 349, 31 January 1991, p. 374.

15. John Maddox, letter to Joan Shenton, 12 February 1991.
16. MRC press release, 15 May 1992.
17. *New York Native*, 15 June 1992.
18. *Sunday Times*, 24 May 1992.
19. *Lancet*, 23 May 1992.
20. *Science*, vol. 251, 22 March 1991, pp. 1422–3.
21. David Sharp, letter to Joan Shenton, 1 July 1992.
22. *Independent*, 20 May 1992.
23. William Waldegrave, answer to written question from George Galloway, House of Commons, 12 May 1993, OPSS Ref: 1992/93/1–0695.
24. Joan Shenton, letters to Andreas Whittam Smith, 21 and 26 May 1992.
25. Sir Gordon Downey, letter to Joan Shenton, 18 June 1992.
26. Simon Jenkins, personal conversation, June 1992.

Chapter 10: AIDS and Africa

1. Kary Mullis interview with Russell Schoch, *Newsweek*, 17 August 1992.
2. Drew Hopkins, *City Week*, 17 October, 1988.
3. Anton Geser and Glen Burbaker, 'AIDS and Africa: An Alternative Hypothesis', unpublished paper, 1988.
4. Celia Farber, 'Out of Africa' parts 1 and 2, *Spin Magazine*, March and April 1993.
5. *AIDS and Africa*, Dispatches, Channel 4, 1993.
6. Kevin de Cock, *British Medical Journal*, vol. 289, 1984, pp. 306–8.
7. Robert Gallo, 'Virus Hunting, AIDS cancer and the human retrovirus', A New Republic Book, Basic Books, (Harper Collins) 1991, pp. 226–8.
8. L.-J. Eales, J. M. Parkin and A. J. Pinching, *Lancet*, vol. 1, 2 May 1987, pp. 999–1002.
9. Jad Adams, *AIDS: The HIV Myth*, Macmillan,1989, p. 179.
10. R. M. Anderson and Robert May, 'Understanding the AIDS Pandemic', *Scientific American*, May 1992.
11. L.-J. Eales, K. E. Nye and A. J. Pinching, *Lancet*, vol. 1, 1988, p. 936.
12. C. Mulder, 'Human virus not from monkeys', *Nature*, vol. 333, 2 June 1988, p. 396.
13. Alan Cantwell, *New African*, October 1994.
14. G. Hunsmann, *British Medical Journal*, vol. 293, 27 September 1986.
15. Dr Felix Konotey Ahulu, 'What is AIDS?', Tetteh-A'Demeno Co., Watford, England, 1989.
16. Richard and Rosalind Chirimuuta, *AIDS, Africa and Racism*, Free Association Books, London, 1989.
17. *Lancet*, 25 July 1987, pp. 206–7.
18. *AIDS and Africa*, Dispatches, Channel 4, programme transcript, 1993.
19. R. M. Anderson, 'The spread of HIV-1 in Africa: sexual contact patterns and the predicted demographic impact of AIDS', *Nature*, vol. 352, 15 August 1991; R. M. Anderson, Lecture, Imperial College, London 'The AIDS Pandemic', 3 November 1992.
20. Charles Geshekter, *New African*, October 1994.

21. *AIDS and Africa*, op. cit.
22. Ibid.
23. Ibid.
24. Ibid.
25. Felix Konotey-Ahulu, *British Medical Journal*, vol. 294, 20 June 1987, pp. 1593–4; O. Kashala et al., *Journal of Infectious Diseases*, vol. 169, February 1994, pp. 296–304; B. L. Bermas, *AIDS Research and Human Retroviruses*, vol. 10, no. 9, 1994; A. D. Harries, *Lancet*, vol. 335, 17 February 1990, pp. 387–90; *Journal of the American Medical Association*, vol. 260, 19 August 1988, p. 260; *New England Journal of Medicine*, vol. 318, 18 February 1988, pp. 448–9. *Lancet*, 28 October 1989, pp. 1023–5; M. Fraziano and V. Colizzi et al., *AIDS Research and Human Retroviruses*, vol. 12, no. 6, 1996, pp. 491–6; Barthel and Wallace, *Sem. Arthrit. Rheumat.*, vol. 23, 1993, pp. 1–7.
26. *Journal of the American Medical Association*, vol. 268, 1992, pp. 1015–17.
27. Alexander Voevodin, *Lancet*, vol. 339, 20 June 1992.
28. Andrew Swai, *Lancet*, 21 October 1989.
29. O. Kashala et al., *Journal of Infectious Diseases*, vol. 169, February 1994, pp. 296–304.
30. *AIDS and Africa*, op. cit.
31. Ibid.
32. Ibid.
33. Ibid.
34. Dr Betty Mpeka, *AIDS and Africa*, op. cit.
35. *AIDS and Africa*, op. cit.
36. Ibid.
37. Ibid.
38. Harvey Bialy, *AIDS and Africa*, op. cit.
39. Ibid.
40. Ibid.
41. Ibid.
42. Peter Duesberg, *Science*, vol. 257, 21 September 1992, p. 1848.
43. Michelle Cochrane, personal conversation.
44. O. Hishida et al., *Lancet*, vol. 340, pp. 971–2.
45. K. M. de Cock et al., *British Medical Journal*, vol. 302, 1991, p. 1206.
46. *AIDS and Africa*, op. cit.
47. Ibid.
48. A. Fauci, *New England Journal of Medicine*, vol. 328, 1993, pp. 429–31.
49. P. Duesberg, *Bio/Technology*, vol. 11, August 1993, pp. 955–6.
50. *AIDS and Africa*, op. cit.
51. Steve Connor, *Sunday Times*, 10 December 1995.

Chapter 11: Diary of an AIDS Dissident

1. Celia Farber, *Diary of an AIDS Dissident*, Meditel Productions, transmitted on Sky News, 29 November 1993, programme transcript.

Notes

2. Peter Duesberg, 'AIDS acquired by drug consumption and other noncontagious risk factors', *Pharmacology and Therapeutics*, vol. 55, 1992, pp. 210–77.
3. *Diary of an AIDS Dissident*, op. cit.
4. Ibid.
5. John Crewdson, 'The great AIDS quest: science under the microscope', *Chicago Tribune*, 19 November 1989.
6. *Science*, vol. 248, 22 June 1990.
7. John Crewdson, 'The great AIDS quest: science under the microscope', op. cit.
8. *Lancet*, 20 January 1990.
9. Robert Gallo, letter to *Nature*, vol. 351, 30 May 1991, p. 358.
10. Steve Connor, *Independent on Sunday*, 2 June 1991.
11. *New York Times*, 31 December 1992.
12. Paul Recer, Associated Press science writer, 30 December 1992.
13. *Lancet*, vol. 431, 3 April 1993.
14. MRC press notice, 2 April 1993.
15. Medical Research Council, PENTA 1 trial, 3 February 1992 (amended 8 December 1992.)
16. *AZT Babies*, Meditel Productions, transmitted on Sky News, June 1993.
17. Ibid.
18. *Diary of an AIDS Dissident*, op. cit.
19. Ibid.
20. Ibid.
21. Ibid.
22. Martin Walker, *Dirty Medicine*, Slingshot Publications, London, 1993
23. *Diary of an AIDS Dissident*, op. cit.
24. Ibid.
25. Ibid.
26. V. I. Avramis et al., *AIDS: Current Science*, vol. 3, 1989, pp. 417–22; J. Balzarini et al., *Journal of Biological Chemistry*, vol. 264, 1989, pp. 6127–33; H.-T. Ho and M. J. M. Hitchcock, *Antimicrobial Agents and Chemotherapy*, vol. 33, 1989, pp. 844–9; M. Mansuri et al., *Antimicrobial Agents and Chemotherapy*, vol. 34, 1990, pp. 637–41; M. J. M. Hitchcock, *Antiviral Chemistry and Chemotherapy*, vol. 2, 1991, pp. 125–32.
27. Graham McKerrow, 'It's time to lift the censorship', *Capital Gay*, August/September 1993.
28. *New York Native*, 13 July 1992.
29. Neville Hodgkinson, *Sunday Times*, 6 June 1993.
30. MRC press notice, 15 September, 1993.
31. SCAM dossier presented to MRC, Meditel archive, 30 November 1993.
32. Medical Research Council, PENTA 1 trial, 3 February 1992 (amended 8 December 1992.)
33. George Galloway, letter to MRC, 29 November 1993.
34. MRC letter to Martin Walker, chairman SCAM, February 1994.
35. Christopher Dunkley, *Financial Times*, 1 December 1993.
36. *Lancet*, vol. 345, 18 February 1995.

Chapter 12: Whatever Happened to AIDS in Haiti?

1. Dennis Altman, AIDS *in the Mind of America*, Anchor Doubleday, New York, 1986; UK edition, AIDS *in the New Puritanism*, Pluto, London, 1986.
2. Randy Shilts, *And the Band Played On*, Penguin, Harmondsworth, 1988.
3. Pape et al., *Am. J. Med. Sci.*, 1986, vol. 291, p. 4.
4. Worth Cooley-Prost, personal communication, March 1996.
5. Ibid.

Chapter 13: Poppers and AIDS: Haemophilia and AIDS

1. I. Quinto, *Bollettino Società Italiana Biologia Sperimentale*, vol. 56, 1980, pp. 816–20; J. Osterloh, *Journal of Analytical Toxicology*, July/August 1984, pp. 164–9.
2. J. Lauritsen and H. Wilson, *Death Rush: Poppers and AIDS*, Pagan Press, New York, 1986.
3. Andrew Moss, 'A case-control study of risk factors for AIDS in San Francisco', presentation to the CDC AIDS Conference in Atlanta, 15 April 1985.
4. I. Quinto, op. cit., J. Osterloh, op. cit.
5. Karl Jorgensen, *New England Journal of Medicine*, 30 September 1982, pp. 1893–4.
6. Harry Haverkos, *Environmental Health Perspectives*, vol. 102, 10 October 1994.
7. *Capital Gay*, 20 August, 1993.
8. *Birmingham Post*, 3 March 1994.
9. Ibid.
10. Stephen Lutener, personal conversation, April 1997.
11. P. Volberding et al., 'Zidovudine in asymptomatic human immunodeficiency virus infection', *New England Journal of Medicine*, vol. 322, no. 14, 5 April 1990.
12. P. Duesberg, 'Immunodeficiency in haemophiliacs with and without HIV', submission to the *Lancet*, 20 August 1992.
13. P. Duesberg, *Pharmac. Ther.*, vol. 55, 1992, pp. 201–77; *Genetica*, vol. 95, 1995, pp. 51–70.
14. Ibid.
15. Centers for Disease Control, *AIDS Surveillance*, year-end edition, 1992.
16. P. Duesberg, 'Immunodeficiency in haemophiliacs with and without HIV', op. cit.
17. Ibid.
18. C. Ludlum, *Lancet*, 28 May 1988.
19. Ibid.
20. Neville Hodgkinson, *Sunday Times*, 22 February 1993.
21. Ibid.
22. Russell Schoch, *California Monthly*, April 1990, p. 9; Steve Heimoff, *Cal Report*, autumn 1991 issue.
23. R. Schoch, *Newsweek*, 17 August 1992
24. Eleni Eleopulos, *Genetica*, vol. 95, 1995, pp. 25–50
25. Ibid.
26. Ibid.

27. Ibid, p. 30.
28. David Raznick, *Reappraising AIDS*, vol. 5, no. 5, March 1997.
29. Eleni Eleopulos, *Genetica*, op. cit.
30. F. Wong-Staal and R. C. Gallo, *Nature*, vol. 317, pp. 395–403.
31. J. Schupback et al., *AIDS*, vol. 6, 1992, pp. 1545–6.
32. L. Kozhemiakin and I. Bondarenko, *Biochimiia*, vol. 57, 1992, pp. 1417–26.
33. H. Barthel and D. Wallace, *Sem. Arthrit. Rheumat.*, vol. 23, 1993, pp. 1–7.
34. Eleni Eleopulos, *Genetica*, op. cit.
35. Ibid.
36. Sarah Darby et al., letter to *Nature*, vol. 377, 7 September 1995.
37. John Maddox, *Nature*, vol. 377, 7 September 1995.
38. MRC press notice, 7 September 1995.
39. Steve Connor, *Independent*, 8 September 1995.
40. Peter Duesberg, letter, *Lancet*, vol. 346, 18 November 1995.
41. Ibid.
42. *Continuum*, vol. 3, no. 3, September/October 1995.
43. *Continuum*, vol. 3, no. 4, November/December 1995.

Chapter 14: Does HIV Exist?

1. Stefan Lanka, 'HIV: reality or artefact?', *Continuum*, vol. 3, no. 1, April/May 1995.
2. E. Eleopulos, 'Is a positive Western blot proof of HIV infection?', *Bio/Technology*, vol. 11, June 1993.
3. Stefan Lanka, 'HIV: reality or artefact?', op. cit.
4. Ibid.
5. A. Hässig et al., 'Stress-induced suppression of the cellular immune reactions. A contribution on the neuroendocrine control of the immune system', Berne Study Group on Nutrition and Immunity, Elisabethenstr 51, CH–3014, Berne, Switzerland, 1995; A. Hässig et al., 'Reflections on the pathogenesis and prevention of AIDS', Berne Study Group on Nutrition and Immunity.
6. A. Fauci, *Journal of Clinical Investigation*, vol. 53, 1974, p. 240.
7. A. Hässig et al., 'Open questions concerning the specificity of anti-HIV antibodies', Berne Study Group on Nutrition and Immunity, May 1996.
8. B. L. Bermas, *AIDS Research and Human Retroviruses*, vol. 10 no. 9, 1994; M. Fraziano and V. Colizzi et al., *AIDS Research and Human Retroviruses*, vol. 12, no. 6, 1996, pp. 491–6.
9. W. Lewis and M. Dalakas, *Nature Medicine*, vol. 1, no. 5, May 1995, pp. 417–22.
10. Gary Pace and Cynthia Leef, 'The Role of Oxidative Stress in HIV Disease', *Free Radical Biology and Medicine*, vol. 19, no. 4, 1995, pp. 523–8.
11. A. Hässig et al., *Schweiz. Zschr. GanzheitsMedizin*, vol. 5, 1990, pp. 234–9.
12. A. Hässig et al., 'Stress-induced suppression of the cellular immune reactions. A contribution on the neuroendocrine control of the immune system', Berne Study Group on Nutrition and Immunity, op cit., 1995; W. X. Liang, K. Stampfli, A. Hässig, 'Ballaststoffe und anti-oxidantien–relevanz fur enstetehung und prävention

Notes

nicht infektiöser zivilizationserkrankungen', *Forschend Komplementarmed*, vol. 2, 1995.

13. A. Hässig et al., 'Suggestions for the prevention of AIDS in HIV carriers', *Schewizerische Zeitschrift fur GanzheitsMedizin*, vol. 4, no. 93, pp. 188–92.
14. E. Eleopulos, 'Is a positive Western blot proof of HIV infection?', op. cit.
15. Valendar Turner, *Continuum*, vol. 3, no. 5, January/February 1996.
16. V. M. Edwards et al., *Am. J. Clin. Pathol.* vol. 91, pp. 75–8.
17. Valendar Turner, *Continuum*, vol. 3, no. 4, p. 20.
18. Philip Mortimer, *Lancet*, vol. 337, 2 February 1991, pp. 286–7.
19. E. Eleopulos, letter, *Lancet*, vol. 347, 20 January 1996.
20. D. S. Burke, *New England Journal of Medicine*, vol. 319, 1988, pp. 961–4.
21. Valendar Turner, *Continuum*, vol. 3, no. 5, January/February 1996.
22. *Journal of the American Medical Association (JAMA)*, 19 August 1988.
23. Eleni Eleopulos, 'Is a positive Western blot proof of HIV infection?', *JAMA*, 19 August 1988; Eleni Eleopulos et al., 'The isolation of HIV: has it really been achieved? The case against', *Continuum*, vol. 4, no. 3, Supplement, September/October 1993.
24. Peter Duesberg, *Continuum*, vol. 4, no. 5, February/March 1997.
25. Ibid.
26. Philip Mortimer, conversation with James Whitehead, April 1996.
27. *Journal of the American Medical Association*, vol. 260, 19 August 1988, p. 260; *New England Journal of Medicine*, vol. 318, 18 February 1988, pp. 448–9; *Lancet*, 28 October 1989, pp. 102–5.
28. Hector Severino, personal interview, July 1996.
29. Fiona Barton, *Mail on Sunday*, 21 April 1996.
30. Alan Bruce, personal communication, 10 July 1997.
31. R. S. Remis, *Canadian Medical Association Journal*, 1990, pp. 1247–54; P. M. Neumann, *J. Acquired Immune Deficiency Syndrome*, 1990, vol. 3, pp. 278–81.
32. Vittorio Colizzi, *AIDS research and human retroviruses*, 1996, vol. 12, pp. 491–6; V. Colizzi et al., personal communication to Eleopulos et al., 1996; personal communication to Shenton, April 1997.
33. Clare Thompson, *Sunday Times Magazine*, 30 June 1996.
34. Ibid.
35. P. Mortimer, 'Towards error free diagnosis: notes on laboratory practice', *PHLS Microbiology Digest*, vol. 9, no. 2, 1992, pp. 61–4.
36. Sheryl Gay Stolberg, 'Despite new AIDS drugs, many still lose the battle', *New York Times*, 22 August 1997.
37. Richard A. Knox, *The Boston Globe*, 25 February 1997.
38. Synapse (University of California at San Francisco student paper), vol. 41, no. 6, 10 October 1996, p. 1.
39. Physicians' Desk Reference, Medical Economics Company, New Jersey, USA, 1997.
40. 'Doctors, new AIDS drug failing', Associated Press, 29 September 1997.
41. Mark Jacobson, *Lancet*, 17 May 1997.
42. Jim Lumb, personal communication, 23 October 1997.
43. 'AIDS Treatment Update', *Issue* 56/7, August/September 1997, pp. 5, 10.
44. Simon Collins, 'Extending the armoury', *Positive Nation*, October 1997, pp. 40–1.
45. John Stevens, 'Taking on the side effects', *Positive Nation*, October 1997, pp. 42–3.

Bibliography

Adams, Jad, *AIDS: The HIV Myth*, Macmillan,1989

Altman, Dennis, *Homosexual Oppression and Liberation*, Plymbridge, Boston, 1993

— AIDS *in the Mind of America*, Anchor Doubleday, New York, 1986; UK edition, AIDS *in the New Puritanism*, Pluto, London, 1986

Callen, Michael, *Surviving* AIDS, Harper & Row, London, September 1990

Chirimuuta, Richard and Rosalind, *AIDS Africa and Racism*, Free Association Books, London, 1989

Duesberg, Peter, *Inventing the AIDS Virus*, Regnery Publishing, Inc., Washington DC, 1996

— *AIDS: Virus or Drug-Induced*, Kluwer Academic Publishers, Netherlands, 1996

Ellison, Bryan J. and P. H. Duesberg, *Why We Will Never Win the War on AIDS*, Inside Story Communications, El Cerrito, California, 1994

Franchi, Fabio and Luigi de Marchi, *AIDS: 'La Grande Truffa'*, SEAM, Rome, 1996

Gallo, Robert, *Virus Hunting: AIDS, Cancer and the Human Retrovirus*, A New Republic Book, Basic Books, Harper Collins, London, 1991

Hodgkinson, Neville, *AIDS: The Failure of Contemporary Science – How a virus that never was deceived the world*, Fourth Estate, London, 1996

Holub, William and Claudia, 'AIDS' . . . *Careful Scientific Scrutiny Provides a Totally Different View*, Life Systems, 174 Bagatelle Road, Melville NY 11747, 1988 (ISBN 0–942494–52–0)

Konotey Ahulu, Felix, *What is AIDS?*, Tetteh-A'Demeno Company, Watford, England, 1989

Kramer, Larry, *Faggots*, Minerva, New York, 1990

Lang, Serge, *Challenges*, Springer Verlag, New York, November 1997

Lauritsen, John, *Poison by Prescription: The AZT Story* (Foreword by Peter Duesberg), Asklepios, New York, 1990 (ISBN 0 943742–06–4)

— *The AIDS War*, Asklepios, New York, 1993 (ISBN 0–943742–08–0)

Lauritsen, John and Hank Wilson, *Death Rush: Poppers and AIDS*, Pagan Press, New York, 1986

Lauritsen, John and Ian Young (eds), *The AIDS Cult: Essays on the Gay Health Crisis*, Asklepios, Provincetown, 1997; Pagan Press, Box 1902, Provincetown, MA 02657–0245

Miller, David J. and Michael Hersen (eds), *Research Fraud in the Behavioural and Biomedical Sciences*, John Wiley, New York/Chichester, 1992 (ISBN 0–471–52068–3)

Paglia, Camille, *Sex, Art, and American Culture*, Viking, London, 1992

Root-Bernstein, Robert, *Rethinking AIDS*, The Free Press, New York, 1993

Bibliography

Schwartz, Joseph, *Creative Moment*, Jonathan Cape, London, 1994

Scott, Andrew, *Pirates of the Cell*, Basil Blackwell, Oxford, revised 1987 (ISBN 0–631–15637–2)

Shilts, Randy, *And the Band Played On*, Penguin, Harmondsworth, 1988

Soda, T. (ed.), Drug-*Induced Sufferings: Medical, Pharmaceutical, and Legal Aspects*, Excerpta Medica, Amsterdam, 1980

Walker, Martin, *Dirty Medicine*, Slingshot Publications, London, 1993

Index

Index

Index

Index

Index

Index

Index

Index

Index

Index